To the amazing women in my life:
My mothers, my grandmothers, my sisters,
my strong and faithful friends.
You inspire me.

Also by Lissa Coffey:

CLOSURE and the Law of Relationship: Endings as New Beginnings

What's Your Dosha, Baby? Discover the Vedic Way for Compatibility in Life and Love

Getting There with Grace: Simple Exercises for Experiencing Joy

Getting There! 9 Ways to Help Your Kids Learn What Matters Most in Life

The Healthy Family Handbook: Natural Remedies for Parents and Children

Freddy Bear's Wakeful Winter

For more information, or to sign up for free newsletters, visit Lissa's websites:

WhatsYourDharma.com
CoffeyTalk.com
WhatsYourDosha.com
PSMeditation.com
CoffeyBuzz.com
FamilyEveryday.com
DoshaDesign.com

Table of Contents

Foreword

Does it surprise you that I first did yoga when I was in college? And that I only did it to impress a girl?

I mean let's be real: you grow up the son of his holiness Deepak Chopra and there's a certain expectation that you're a born and bred yogi, that you're vegan straight out of the womb, and that you're an instinctive master of the seven spiritual laws from conception.

Alas...

Even if I haven't evolved that much in the last thirty years or so, Yoga has. I remember growing up in Boston, Massachusetts when my father first started talking about it as a practical way to reduce stress, lessen chronic fatigue, enhance strength and flexibility - even as way of treating indigestion and other health related issues. Most people smirked at these alien ideas, dismissing yoga as a fringe practice of eastern occultists. Oh how things have changed. Today, according to Google maps, there are over a dozen yoga studios within a three-mile radius of my house. And by the way, you can select from power yoga, hot yoga, dance yoga and all sorts of other trademarked forms of yoga. On the contrary, nowadays fringe groups of eastern occultists are enraged that they don't get credit for yoga which is often regarded as just another trendy exercise regimen in a long line of Taibo, pilates, spinning and other assorted aerobic routines.

Yoga is just one of various eastern vernacular that has moved from the fringe to the mainstream. *Karma, mantra, Guru,* and *dharma* are some others that spring to mind. All of these words, these *ideas,* are rich in substance, tradition, ritual, and meaning. In the modern world – err popular western culture – they've become twitter terms and motivational monikers for a culture often mired in chaos and in desperate search for feel good moments. As a consequence, what gets lost in the lore of this self-help scene is the deeper resonance of these ideas and how they practically connect with us in our modern lives.

In other words, I want to live and work in the modern world, but I have questions about the deeper meaning and purpose of my life at the same time. I want to be successful at what I do, see that result in material abundance and prosperity, but learn how not to have my sense of self-worth be dependent on that materialism. I want to be engaged in the world and those closest to me, but be detached and spiritually liberated too.

We live in conflicting times. The world is getting flatter, smaller, and more connected at a pace more rapid than we can even conceive. We're socially networked ad infinitem, and yet we're more lost than ever. Why? Because modern culture tells us that you're one or the other, sacred or profane, divine or diabolical, jacked in or zoned out, even though in truth most of us are a bit of cut and paste of all of the above.

So how do we make sense of it all? We find teachers that have spent their lives studying and *living* the wisdom traditions of ancient cultures. These are people who take pride in their imperfection, teachers who don't have spiritual prefixes or devoted posses. These are real people living in the real world dealing with real issues and finding real solutions. These are people like Lissa Coffey who have devoted their lives to the search for fulfillment and happiness, who say with pride that it's not the secrets they've found that are their greatest revelation, but the gypsy-like search for them that comprises the secrets themselves.

How do I know? Because I just finished reading the galley copy of the book you're holding in your hands right now. Because I feel smarter and happier and more equipped for the road ahead of me that will surely be full of potholes, unexpected twists and turns, and wild variable along the way. And because well, I happen to know my way around spiritual teachers.

And oh by the way, that yoga class to impress the girl? That girl is my wife now so I guess I have kind of evolved. A little bit, anyway.

Gotham Chopra

Introduction

"Dharma" is a Sanskrit word meaning "purpose." Vedic Sanskrit is likely the world's oldest language, dating back as early as 1500 BC. In Sanskrit, each word, and each syllable, has layers of meaning. Dharma actually has 16 different translations, one of which means teachings, or lessons. This seems appropriate because in many ways, our life's purpose is our lesson, and vice-versa. We each come to feel at some point in our lives that there is something important for us to do, or learn, or experience. We understand that there has to be something more than just living day to day. Another meaning of dharma is truth. As we grow in awareness, we seek to know truth, that deeper meaning to life, and what it is all about. We seek our dharma, to fulfill our purpose, to somehow have our lives make sense in the context of everything that is going on in the world.

> "Everything—a horse, a vine—is created for some duty...For what task, then, were you yourself created? A man's true delight is to do the things he was made for. "
>
> -Marcus Aurelius

When we talk about "purpose" it is clear that we each have our individual purpose – a reason why we're here on this planet in this specific place and time – and that's up to each of us to figure out for ourselves. And then generally, we all have the same purpose, or dharma, which is three-fold:

1. To learn and grow. It seems to be our natural instinct to progress in this way. We can't grow backwards! We look for opportunities to better ourselves, and we find them all around us. We practice behaviors that help us to understand who we are. We look within. Journaling is an example of a way for us to keep track of our thoughts, dreams and desires. It's also a way that we can look back and see how far we've come. Spiritual growth is a strong desire, one that propels us forward.

2. To express ourselves and our unique gifts. We are not meant to sit in a shadow and be quiet. We have something to say, both literally and figuratively. So, just what are these unique gifts that we have to share with the world? It's personal for each one of us. It takes all of us, and all of our varied and diverse talents, to make this world function.

3. To help each other. Many times this goes really well with the second part, and we can use our talent to help others. For example, my mother loves to crochet, and she can whip up

a blanket in no time at all. She and a group of her friends knit and crochet items for children in hospitals. They also make hats and booties for our soldiers to send over in care packages. Helping feels good. And we have so many chances everyday to really make a difference in the world.

We are all connected, and we are here to help each other learn and grow. That's the Law of Relationship. But just exactly *how* do we do that? How do we know what our individual purpose is? How do we know what our unique talents are? How can we make best use of our time and energy so that we are doing something worthwhile with our lives?

> *"What we must decide is perhaps how we are valuable, rather than how valuable we are."*
>
> -F. Scott Fitzgerald

Vedanta, based on the sacred scriptures of India, is likely the world's most ancient religion, and the religion from which all others were born. Because of the connection that we all share, Vedanta recognizes the "oneness" of all beings. And because we have this connection not only with each other, but with God, the Universe, Spirit, Brahman or whatever name we choose to use for this Divine Energy that runs through us and all around us, Vedanta says that each soul is divine. Our main objective in life is to realize our divinity, and Vedanta explains that not only is it possible for us to do this, it is indeed inevitable.

Vedanta also declares that all religious philosophies share the same basic truths about our relationships, and about God. The Rig Veda, a text that is thousands of years old, says: *"Truth is one, sages call it by various names."* Though each religion may offer a different approach, each is valid. Any seeming conflicts in messaging are caused by dogma and politics. When we look closely at the spiritual truth, we find all that there really is in common amongst the world's religions. For this reason, I have also included throughout this book wisdom from a variety of different religions, cultures, and times in history to support the inherent message.

In the west, we think of yoga primarily as a form of exercise. Although physical postures make up one branch of this philosophy, yoga in general is so much more. The Sanskrit word "yoga" means to yoke, or to unite. The purpose of yoga is to experience the connection we have with the Divine. In Vedanta there are four different yogas, or spiritual practices, to help us to accomplish this feeling of connection. The yogas can be practiced individually or in combination, as each one balances and strengthens the others. Each one is a kind of path to discovering our divinity. We can map out our own course using our particular interests and strengths, based on the direction that Vedanta provides us.

The four yoga paths could be thought of as bridges, bringing us from a limited understanding of who we think we are, to the greater understanding of who we really are. These paths help us to be aware of, and express, our purpose, our dharma, through love, work, knowledge and meditation. Yes, we can, and do, learn through each of these paths. However our personalities will guide us more toward one path or another, so that we can focus our attention and use the strengths we have to understand these spiritual concepts in a way that makes sense to us.

The path itself is our purpose, or our dharma. We tend to think that there is some end destination waiting for us somewhere. But the truth is, we are where we are, in this moment, in this place and time, and the best we can do is to be fully present. Every step we take, every choice we make, holds meaning and creates space for us to go again. We learn all along the way. It's not like we have to "get there" and then we have an epiphany where we suddenly understand, where our dharma is clear and all the answers are presented to us. We live our dharma. We express our dharma with everything we think, say, and do.

Bhakti Yoga is the path of love and devotion. Bhakti is the love of all creation. It is about loving what is, without expectation. Through our relationships with people we can experience a greater awareness. There is a power, a positive energy that comes with love, that we can utilize for our spiritual growth. Vedanta explains that our love for others is unselfish and without motive when we can see the spirit within them. It is this spirit whom we truly love. So we can learn to look beyond the limiting qualities of the human to the transcendent qualities of the divine, and fully experience love heart to heart. Love is available to all of us, and it is an irresistible force! We spend our time, and emotions, developing a kind of bond with a person. Our energy goes into these connections, along with our emotions, our hopes, and our human vulnerabilities. With Bhakti Yoga, we learn through our relationships, and through our primary relationship, which is with ourselves.

Karma Yoga is the path of work, or the path of service. This is work without attachment to the end result. Rather than working for a paycheck, it is performing the work we do as a spiritual offering. Karma Yoga teaches us that working merely for money, or promotions, or praise, leads us to disappointment, because we can never meet all of our expectations; it is never "enough." However, working as a service to ourselves and to others, allows us to experience spirit in everything we do. We are connected to our work, and the actions become effortless. We feel that God is working through us, and this gives us both energy and peace of mind. We learn to love what we do.

Jnana Yoga is the path of knowledge. This is knowledge in the higher sense, knowing who we are, and being aware of our relationship, our connection, with God. Knowing is different than believing, it uses reasoning to help us shed the veil of illusion. Vedanta gives us tools to achieve this through affirmations that help to remind us of what is real, and to see the truth. Jnana Yoga teaches to become more discerning, recognizing the difference between what is temporary and what is eternal, so that we understand that we are pure, perfect, and free.

We are all students, and we are all teachers. Our learning never ends. It is through this process of learning that we grow both intellectually and spiritually. We come to understand that the only thing we really take with us from this life experience is the wisdom that we garner. We learn to love what we learn and also the process of learning itself.

Raja Yoga is the path of meditation. By stilling the mind through meditation, we can experience more of our true selves. Raja Yoga explains that we need to settle down the mind, which is constantly stirred up with thoughts just as a lake is muddied through activity. When the lake settles down, the water becomes crystal clear, and so it is with our mind. This tranquil state of mind lets us think more clearly, and to see what is important in life. Through meditation we have direct experience of our connection with God. And Vedanta teaches us that we can integrate this experience into all aspects of our life. We don't have to live in an ashram or renounce our worldly belongings. Our spiritual self is our *true* self and we can operate in society more effectively and efficiently when we understand this. We learn to love who we are.

"Chanting is no more holy than listening to the murmur of a stream, counting prayer beads no more sacred than simply breathing, religious robes no more spiritual than work clothes."

–Lao-tsu

There is wisdom to be gained from each of these paths. They all end up taking us to the same place, to the recognition of our union with the divine, to the discovery of our dharma, our purpose. The paths work in harmony with one another. We find that there are aspects of each path that we relate to. Yet quite often one of these paths will resonate with particular individuals more than the others. One will seem to offer a more clear direction, a more personal journey. To help you determine which path might be the one most productive for you, I've come up with a short Dharma quiz. This is not scientific, there are no right or wrong answers; this is just for your own personal inventory. It's another way of getting to know yourself better.

The Dharma Quiz

For the following questions, circle the answer that you like the most.

1. Which type of show are you most likely to download?

   a. Romance
   b. documentary
   c. mystery or instructional
   d. nature

2. You have the afternoon off, how do you prefer to spend your time?

   a. hanging out with my honey
   b. volunteering for my favorite charitable organization
   c. browsing the bookstore
   d. quiet time alone

3. Time to travel, where do you prefer to go?

    a. Back to my hometown for a family reunion
    b. Africa to help build schools
    c. Europe to visit museums
    d. India on a meditation retreat

4. You're going to a party, how do you participate?

    a. I bring a picture frame for the hostess
    b. I help clean up afterwards
    c. I share stories with the other guests
    d. I play music for the other guests

5. When you were 7 years old, what did you want to be when you grew up?

    a. doctor/nurse/veterinarian/parent
    b. chef/builder/president/fireman/athlete
    c. teacher/lawyer/detective/scientist
    d. pilot/dancer/forest ranger/artist

6. A friend is not feeling well, how do you respond?

    a. I go visit and bring flowers
    b. I drop off homemade chicken soup
    c. I research remedies online
    d. I light a candle and send prayers

7. You win a $100 cash prize, how do you spend it?

   a. I buy a gift for someone I love
   b. I make a donation to a non-profit organization
   c. I sign up for a class I've wanted to take
   d. I buy noise-canceling headphones

8. What song best describes your lifestyle?

   a. Love Makes the World Go Round
   b. Heal The World
   c. Learn to Live
   d. Imagine

9. Which animal best fits your personality?

   a. kitten
   b. horse
   c. dolphin
   d. swan

10. If you could go back in time, whom would you most like to have dinner with?

    a. A long lost relative
    b. Eleanor Roosevelt
    c. Albert Einstein
    d. The Buddha

11. What was your favorite part of your school days?

    a. Making friends
    b. Going to scouts/student council/sports
    c. Learning new things
    d. art/band/choir

12. How do you celebrate your birthday?

    a. Invite family over
    b. Bring a cake to the office
    c. Go to a play or to hear a speaker
    d. Go to a spa

13. Which quote speaks to you the most?

    a. "Love is the central flame of the universe, nay, the very fire itself." -Ernest Holmes
    b. "Serve self you serve society, Serve society serve yourself." - Ralph Waldo Emerson
    c. "I am still learning." -Michelangelo
    d. "Speak, move, act in peace, as if you were in prayer. In truth, this is prayer." -Francis de S. Fenelon

Now add up the letters that you circled and write the total here:

A_____ B_____ C_____ D_____

If you have mostly "A" answers, then the path that likely speaks most strongly to you is Bhakti Yoga, the path of LOVE.

If you have mostly "B" answers, then the path that fits your personality the most is likely Karma Yoga, the path of WORK.

If you have mostly "C" answers, then the path that is likely to benefit you the most is Jnana Yoga, the path of KNOWLEDGE.

If you have mostly "D" answers, then the path you are drawn to the most is likely to be Raja Yoga, the path of MEDITATION.

You may choose to read the section on your particular path first, and if you do then definitely go back and read about the other paths, because there are things that apply to everyone in each discipline, and lessons for us to learn as we study each one.

All paths lead to the same destination. In Vedanta that destination is said to be an awareness of our union with the Divine. We can see this as a deeper understanding of ourselves, and a greater wisdom that comes from experiencing our purpose. We learn to enjoy our lives, and embrace our dharma.

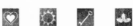

BHAKTI YOGA
The Path of Love

BHAKTI YOGA
The Path of Love

"The state of love is the state of grace."

-N. Sri Ram

LOVE AND DEVOTION

Bhakti Yoga is the path of love and devotion. One who practices bhakti is known as a bhakti-yogi, or a bhakta. The ongoing theme of bhakti yoga is the intense, true, complete, pure, never-ending love of God. The bhakta's constant thought is of loving God. Of the four yogas, bhakti is the most easily accessible to us because we all understand what love is. But do we really?

Love is the most basic human emotion. A person who is attracted to the path of love tends to be someone who follows his or her heart. This is a person who feels emotions deeply, who wears their heart on their sleeve. The heart is strong, and resilient. And the heart is smart; it recognizes truth! When there is a discrepancy between what we feel in our heart and what we know in our head, we often find that our heart knows best. It doesn't steer us wrong. With the heart, we can find inspiration. It has often been said that God speaks to us through the heart. A bhakta values people, and relationships above all else. Love is the priority here; love is what really matters, especially love for God.

If you find that you are a bhakta, then your purpose, your dharma, is to love, and to learn through loving. Recognize that love is strong; it is powerful. Much can be accomplished with love.

LOVE IS

Love can be misconstrued when a person, or a group of people, loves one thing, or one person, or one ideal, in such a way that they hate every other ideal. This is not true love; this is not Bhakti. Practicing Bhakti means loving everyone, and everything, because the bhakta sees God in all of it, as all of it. No conditions, no judgments, and no exceptions. Bhakti, and the Indian philosophy behind it, Vedanta, accepts the practice of all religions, because ultimately the goal is to experience our union with the Divine. In

Vedanta, all paths are valid, have merit and are to be respected and revered. Bhakti is the path that shows us how to experience divine love in our own hearts, at all times. We start right where we are.

THE LANGUAGE OF BHAKTI

There are many times when, as humans, we feel an emotion and there are just no words. We are limited by our language, and by our definitions of words, which are run through our personal filters. How do we describe love? How do we explain God? How do we sum up the Universe? Especially today, when attention spans are short and twitter limits us to 140 characters! A Shakespearean sonnet just won't do. Yet some of the Indian sages have come up with terms to help us understand the experience of divine love. This is something we can relate to because we all have had these kinds of relationships in our lives.

1. **Santa**: peaceful loving. This is love that is calm, and easy. It moves slowly. It is not driven by fire or intensity, but it is steady.

2. **Dasya**: loving God as a master. This is love where a person thinks of himself as a servant to God. He is faithful in his service to the Divine.

3. **Sakhya**: loving God as a friend. In friendship there is a kind of equality, a give and take, a

flow of energy between the two friends. This is the kind of love where we see God as our friend, by our side to share secrets with, to play with.

4. **Vatsalya**: loving God as our child. When we think about how powerful God is, it leaves us in a state of awe. But love has no awe attached to it. Parents do not expect anything of their little children, they don't ask anything of them. They give love to the child without demands or expectations. They don't require any favors in return. In Christianity, we see vatsalya through the image of the Baby Jesus. In Hinduism, this is expressed through the image of the Baby Krishna. Children are pure, and completely lovable.

5. **Madhura**: loving God as our beloved. This is the "madly in love" kind of love. This is the love that we experience as humans most intensely, where we just can't get enough of the other person. The poet Rumi expresses madhura so well in his writings. For example:

> *The minute I heard my first love story*
> *I started looking for you, not knowing*
> *How blind that was.*
> *Lovers don't finally meet somewhere.*
> *They're in each other all along.*

There are many names for God. Each religion has its own vocabulary, and I don't want to list some and end up inadvertently leaving out others. To keep things simple I will use the word God, or the Divine, throughout the book, but you may substitute any name or phrase that works with your background and belief system. The bhakta worships God as a Personal God. When we personalize God, and give "Him" or "Her" a kind of persona. It makes it easier for us to feel the emotion of love because we understand what it feels like to love a person. The huge concept of God as the All-knowing, All-merciful, Eternal, Omnipotent, Omnipresent, is a lot to grasp. So bringing God into a kind of natural form helps us to establish a personal relationship with Him, or Her, or however we choose to address God. The Universe is vast, it is difficult to comprehend how much so. But we can grasp the concept of the earth, the continents, the countries, and on down to our very own community and home. In personalizing God we bring God nearer to us, making God more relatable. The understanding is there, that this personalization is of our own making to suit our human perception.

In our Western culture it is easy for us to be distracted, or to be drawn to the many material things that are available to us. We may desire a car, for example, and say "I love that car!" But this is love misdirected. We can appreciate the car for its functionality, or the beauty of its design. But it is not the car that the bhakta loves. The bhakta loves God. We can see God in the creative process of the car, in the miracle of the machinery, in so many aspects that brought the vehicle into being. But a car is a car. As every material thing, it is impermanent and impersonal. We may feel temporary happiness driving around in a new car, but that will indeed fade. There is no substitute for the bliss that loving God brings. Swami Vivekananda says that with Bhakti we learn that "the eternal interests of the soul are of much higher value than the fleeting interests of this mundane life."

The bhakta only wants to hold love in the heart. Everything else is meaningless. To the bhakta, money is just a tool. When used with love, when used to help others, it can be wonderful. The bhakta is not attached to money, or to any material things, so he gives it freely. To the bhakta, everything pales compared with supreme devotion, so it is easy to cast aside anything that is not love. Whatever emotions come up are directed toward God. It is okay to be angry with God, to feel any emotions and to express them, because there is nothing to struggle against. God is not to be feared, because God does not punish. Love is sweet, gentle, and natural. We can control and direct our passions. We can be more passionate about our spiritual growth!

To the bhakta, love is the only thing that is truly real, and that can bring any satisfaction. With Bhakti Yoga, we learn how to love just for the sake of loving, because it is right and good to love. There is no agenda for our love. We don't love with the expectation that this will get us into heaven, or that wealth will be attracted to us. The bhakta loves because God is love. Wherever love is present, God is present.

"Dear friends, let us love one another, for love comes from God. Everyone who loves has been born of God and knows God."

1 John 4:7

LOVE THE HIGHEST

Bhakti Yoga continually reminds us to "Love the Highest." When all of our human desire for what is new, beautiful or fun is directed instead toward God we experience the greatest delight. When we stand in awe at the stars in the sky, we are reminded of the beauty of the Divine. This beauty is present in all of nature, expressing itself, we only have to notice to feel it.

It is not our purpose to become each other; it is to recognize each other, to learn to see the other and honor him for what he is.

–Hermann Hesse

There are so many songs that talk about love in terms of "desire" and "fire." Love is like a flame that burns bright within each of us. And like fire, when it is controlled it can be directed towards positive uses. A fire can be used to warm us up, or to cook a meal. But when raging out of control it can destroy a home, or a forest. Bhakti Yoga reminds us to always direct our love towards the highest aim, to love God. Love of money, love of possessions, or prestige is misdirected love. Misdirected love can be destructive, leading to heartache and pain. Those who have not embraced Bhakti may feel joy when they receive money, but that joy is fleeting, just as the money is. It comes and it goes. But true love, Bhakti is eternal, and will sustain us.

RELATIONSHIPS

The bhakta understands that even when people come and go, love remains. Because the real love is the love for God, and that never goes away, it never dies. Relationships with people change, but the relationship with God does not. Our relationships provide wonderful opportunities for spiritual growth. We have the relationships we have for a reason. In most cases, the relationship that we are aware of first when we come into this lifetime is the relationship we have with our parents. Every person enters in his own circumstances. Whether we later perceive those circumstances to be positive or negative, the truth is that all circumstances are neutral. Happiness is not a function of our circumstances. We can learn and grow and become closer to God whether we are born in luxury or poverty, in a home filled with delight, or a home filled with strife.

One of the Sanskrit names for God is "Hari," which means "one who attracts all things." We are attracted to the stars, we love the stars, and we see God in the stars. When it comes to a person, the same thing happens. It is the spirit behind the eyes, the God within that attracts us. Bhakti Yoga says that it is the God within that person who we truly love, whether we realize it or not. We're all just walking around as God in disguise, wearing all sorts of different costumes. To the bhakta, every face is the face of God, of Hari.

When I think of unconditional love, and how that presented itself to me at a young age, I think about my grandmother. This woman, although she may not have known the word, was definitely a bhakta.

My grandmother, who left her home and family in Croatia to come to the United States to marry my grandfather, poured love into everything she did. She cooked with love, and loved to feed her children and grandchildren. I remember so many times sitting around her kitchen table, eating her homemade apple strudel, or alphabet soup, and the warmth I felt just being in a place where I knew I was totally welcomed and loved. Her garden was the joy of the neighborhood. She spent hours tending to every plant, giving it love, encouraging it to grow. And you could just see how the flowers responded; they were absolutely glorious! My grandmother saw God in her garden, in her kitchen, in her grandchildren, in her neighbors. Her life was filled with love. Even when she lost her daughter, and then her husband, she was never bitter, she never lost her faith or her love for God. I am so grateful to have had my grandmother and her wonderful example of love in my life. Even though she is not physically with me anymore, I will always carry her love with me. We are still connected.

Many years after my grandmother passed away, I went to see Amma, who is known the "hugging saint." Amma travels the world and hundreds of people line up to see her everywhere she goes. I waited patiently, with all the other people, to see her. When I finally got my hug, the first thought that came to my mind was of my grandmother. It was that same unconditional, warm, loving embrace. It brought tears to my eyes. My heart was overflowing with love. "Amma" is the Sanskrit word for "Mother," and this saint was so named because she loves everyone as her own children. Amma is an example of a Bhakti Yogi. She says: "*An actor takes many roles, but he remains the same. God is like this. Different are His names and forms, but He is the One behind all.*" Amma sees God in everyone, and loves God within everyone. You can feel it in her hugs.

Mother Teresa is another example of a Bhakti Yogi. She gave so much love and care to the most poor, most needy people in Calcutta. She said: "*It's not how much we give, but how much love we put into giving.*" The conditions this brave woman faced in India were rough, to say the least. She constantly dealt with the poverty, and illness in the area, and there was what seemed to be an ever-growing population of people who needed her. When asked how she did it, Mother Teresa would explain that she was so in love with God, and that she could see God within each and every person, that she just had to help. There was nothing else she could do.

Mother Teresa exemplifies compassion. In Pali and Sanskrit the term for compassion is "karuna" and this is an important part of the spiritual path. In Buddhism, loving and kindness go hand-in-hand with one word: "metta." The Pali commentaries explain the difference between karuṇa and metta in the following complementary way: Karuna is the desire to remove harm and suffering from others; while metta is the desire to bring about the happiness and well-being of others.

HOW TO LEARN BHAKTI

The bhakta learns best from people. We are all students, and we are all teachers. We're here to help each other learn and grow. There are things we can't learn from books, we need to experience them ourselves. Love is one of those things. Reading about love and what it feels like to love, and actually feeling love for someone are two completely different experiences.

Each relationship we have has a purpose to it. We can learn from our relationships, and from the people in our lives. There are no accidents, no coincidences. There is an old saying that goes: when the student is ready, the teacher will appear. Sometimes we seek out this teacher, we because we really want to learn. This can be in a formal setting like a classroom, or an office. Or it could be that circumstances present themselves where someone comes into our lives and brings with them all of these opportunities for us to learn. It's up to us to pay attention.

As teachers, it is important that we live our lives by example. Teach love by being loving, and lovable. Practice what has been learned throughout a lifetime by being kind and considerate of others. We never know what impression we are making on those around us, so be ever mindful.

Ellen DeGeneres is known as one of the nicest celebrities in Hollywood. She is a vegan, and she works tirelessly raising funds for several charities as well as giving of her own money. She loves animals. On her talk show, she is warm and open, and always makes her guests as well as her audience feel as if they are her friends. When the topic of bullying became a big issue and was in the news with stories about teen suicides, Ellen responded. She responded with love and compassion. Having someone who understood, and who could relate, and who cared, speak out about this made a big impact and helped the cause immensely. Now, Ellen ends every one of her shows with this tagline: "Be kind to one another." That statement is so simple, and yet so powerful because it is filled with love. Ellen doesn't do this for money, or for fame. She does this because she genuinely cares. This is one way that she expresses love for the community that she serves. And she is walking her talk. She isn't asking people to be kind and then not doing it herself! She is demonstrating kindness every day. Ellen is a bhakta, and a wonderful teacher.

The way you get meaning into your life is to devote yourself to loving others, devote yourself to your community around you, and devote yourself to creating something that gives you purpose and meaning. - Mitch Albom

QUALITIES TO HELP THE LEARNING PROCESS

As a student of any of the yogas, there are three qualities that help with the learning process. The first is purity. This means purity in thought, word and also action. Our thoughts must be pure, because what we think is what we are saying to ourselves, and we need to love and respect ourselves. We must be mindful of what we say to other people, because words can be as harmful as violence, or they can be as healing as medicine. We must also be aware of the impact that our actions have on others. Take every opportunity to help those in need.

The second quality that helps us to learn is a hunger for knowledge. When we want something badly enough we go after it, and we get it. When we want to be a bhakta, we look for teachers, we listen, we read, we practice kindness and demonstrate love at all times, with all of our heart.

And the third quality that helps us in our quest is perseverance. We can't give up. We need to always strive to be better, to overcome challenges and obstacles, and to keep going no matter what.

> *"The purity of life is the highest and most authentic art to follow."*
>
> – *Mahatma Gandhi*

To learn Bhakti, we need to really just dive in. A great teacher, Bhagavan Ramakrishna would often tell a story that applies here. I'm going to call it "Eat the Mango!" A group of students set out to learn about mangos and went to visit a mango orchard. Many of them examined the trees, counted the leaves and the branches, looked at the color and size of the various mangoes. They wrote things down and compared notes. But one student was not interested in any of that. Instead he peeled a mango and ate it. Juice dripped down his chin and he smiled. If you want to know the mango, eat the mango. This is a bhakta. A bhakta doesn't need to know someone's name to love that person. She doesn't need to know a person's age, or hometown. She can love a person just by looking in his eyes and recognizing the divinity within.

You can't buy a certificate, hang it on your wall, and call yourself a Bhakti Yogi. To know Bhakti, you have to love.

HOW TO LIVE BHAKTI

The Vedanta Sutras gives us some tips for how we can nurture Bhakti within ourselves. Bhagavan Ramanuja, one of the great Indian sages, explained that there are certain qualities we can develop to become a bhakta, and among those are: discrimination, controlling the passions, purity, strength and suppression of excessiveness. Let's look at each one of these practices individually.

DISCRIMINATION

The Sanskrit word for discrimination is "viveka." Discrimination is basically making good decisions. It's looking at options and choosing which is the best for us, mentally, spiritually, and physically. Food is just one example of this. We know that there are certain foods that are better for us than others. We need to choose healthy foods, foods that are fresh and filled with vitamins to meet the needs of our body. It takes a certain maturity and discrimination when grocery shopping to read the labels, and understand what the ingredients are and how they affect us. There's also the food that we take into our minds, what we read, the movies we watch, the music we listen to. Is this "food" benefiting us or is it just "junk food?" We need to be discerning, and think about what we are taking in.

We also need to think about what words and conversations we are taking in, and keep company with like-minded people. Sangha is a Sanskrit word that means a gathering. When we gather with people who also want to grow spiritually, we lift ourselves up and we elevate our spirits. We have the choice of where we spend our time, and with whom we spend our time, so choose wisely.

CONTROLLING THE PASSIONS

Controlling the passions means reigning in our senses. We might crave the double chocolate cupcakes, but do we take a bite, or do we scarf down a dozen of them? We don't have to deny our passions, but we do have to temper them with some common sense. Bhakti is love; it's not lust. Rather than thinking, "I LOVE those cupcakes," and indulging our sense of taste, we can think: "I love how God is present in all things." Think about the love that went into the making of the cupcakes, someone spent the time and took care to make them. Look at how beautiful they are, and think about the artistry that went into the decorating of them. We can appreciate the cupcakes for what they are, and consider the whole package, including the calories! Controlling our passion helps us to be discerning. We might choose to recognize the deliciousness of the cupcake, but eat an apple instead. And we can love the apple, too, for so many reasons.

PURITY

Purity goes along these same lines. We keep our body pure with what we eat, and with cleansing it, knowing that this body is the temple through which we experience love. Purity is also an internal process. This means being honest, and kind. It means watching our words and actions, so that we don't harm others, or ourselves.

Purity means forgiveness, not holding on to grudges or grievances. Forgiveness does not condone any behavior – it is releasing attachment to the past. It is freeing oneself from the pain and bitterness that comes with holding on to something we need to let go of. It is knowing that other people are doing the best that they can at any given moment. When the mind is pure we understand that love is ever present and ever abundant, so there is no reason to be jealous of anyone. Love is our priority, and love is our goal, so power, fame, and material wealth are not anything to envy. Purity means that thoughts of revenge or injury to others never cross our mind. We are considerate and respectful of all living beings. The bible says:

> *"Blessed are the pure in heart, for they shall see God."*

> *- Matthew 5:8*

The bhakta understands that we need to be not just tolerant of our differences, but accepting of them.

Wherever we are in the world, we share the same sun. In one place it may be shining in a bright blue sky, in another place it might be hidden behind clouds. People in those various places would describe the sun in a variety of different ways, and yet, it is all the same sun, it is all the truth. When we have this purity of thought, we find that there is no reason to debate, no reason to argue. We can allow for different points of view knowing that the truth is always there. The Bhagavad Gita says:

> *"If you see the soul in every living being, you see truly. If you see immortality in the heart of every mortal being, you see truly."*

Strength

Strength is also important in cultivating Bhakti in our lives. We have to exercise our bodies to be strong, and exercise our mind to be strong as well. Through the five senses, which we have courtesy of the body, we experience the world. The longer we have on this earth, the more opportunity we have to learn lessons, to become wise, to grow in our awareness. We have to take care of ourselves to allow ourselves these opportunities. A strong mind is one that can recognize difficulties and deal with them appropriately. Being strong does not mean overpowering another person; that is not the purpose of strength. Ahimsa is a Sanskrit word meaning "non-violence." Words and attitudes can be destructive weapons, or they can be tools to heal. Bhakti shows us that when we harm another, we harm ourselves, because we are all connected, we are all one.

> *"Nonviolence is the greatest force at the disposal of mankind. It is mightier than the mightiest weapon of destruction devised by the ingenuity of man."*
>
> *—Mahatma Gandhi*

A strong mind doesn't see failure, it sees challenges, and it sees opportunities for growth. When we are strong we know that we can overcome any difficulty that comes our way. We can be optimistic, and cheerful, and we can persevere through trying times.

AVOID EXCESS

Excess is to be avoided. We need to strive for balance, for harmony, for equilibrium. Joy is wonderful, but too much of it distracts us from things that are important in life. Too much grief is also a distraction. We can't indulge our emotions to excess any more than we can indulge our senses to extreme. We need to strive for steadiness, for peace of mind. There are times to be serious, and times to have fun. We can do either of these things without going overboard. In Buddhism, this concept is described as "the middle way," a path between the extremes of austerities and sensual indulgence. The Buddha proclaimed that this path led to liberation, to enlightenment.

Bhakti Yoga says that liberation is a return to love, re-alizing the bliss that is within and around each one of us. It is freedom from the miseries of life; it is a state of joy and a feeling of blessedness. The Sanskrit word for bliss is "ananda." In the Upanishads it says:

> *"from bliss, verily, are these beings born; by bliss, when born, do they live; into bliss, at the time of dis-solution, do they enter, do they merge."*

> *–Taittiriya Upanishad 3.6.1.*

There is a mantra, a short prayer that in Sanskrit is: Sat Chit Ananda. It means, truth, (or also knowing-ness), peace, bliss (or also love). The bhakta medi-tates on this phrase as a reminder of the inner peace that comes with the awareness and knowing of bliss.

The opposite of liberation is bondage. Bhakti Yoga says that this comes from selfishness. It comes from designating "I, me, and mine." The bhakta knows that there is no bliss to be found in material objects. There is no point in hoarding, in accumulating. We don't need any thing in excess. All bliss is found in love, in God. We free ourselves by giving, by sharing, because none of it belongs to us anyway.

> *"Our responsibility is no longer to acquire, but to be."*

> *–Rabindranath Tagore*

LIVING LIFE IN LOVE

Bhakti Yoga shows us that we can live our lives with the constant feeling of being in love. It can be love as a giddy crush, or passionate longing, or a loyal friend or all these things and more at the same time. Whatever the relationship analogy, we recognize true love when it is not the least bit selfish. That is because love gives, love doesn't take away. There is no bargaining or bartering with love because love does not ask for anything in return. There is no ulterior motive, there is just love for the sake of love. The bhakta does not ask anything of God, and does not expect anything from God. God is love itself, and the bhakta loves for the sake of love.

To be a bhakta, when we give love, we need to give without any expectations. That means that we can love without needing to be loved back, without needing to be thanked, without any expectation of any kind of reciprocation, and still feel fulfilled. A bhakta loves "as is." There is no trying to change someone. There is no manipulation. The bhakta knows that everyone and everything is exactly how it should be, and that is perfect.

The other way we can recognize true love is that there is no fear. Love and fear cannot occupy the same space. A Course in Miracles teaches that there are really only two things in life: love and fear. Fear is merely the absence of love, so really, there is only love. The analogy is that there is really only light and dark, and darkness is the absence of light. The bible echoes this same theme:

"There is no fear in love, but perfect love casts out fear."

- *1 John 4:18.*

The bhakta does not interpret God as punishing or rewarding. God is pure love, and how could we fear love?

In Bhakti Yoga, the ultimate realization is the love, the one who loves, and the one who is loved, are all one. To the bhakta, when this is understood we know the truth, we are in our dharma.

EXPRESSIONS OF BHAKTI YOGA

We see Bhakti Yoga out in the world in many different shapes and forms. The doctor, who takes the oath to "first do no harm" is practicing Bhakti. When the surgeon is performing an operation, he or she is seeing the body in terms of its universal characteristics. They know how an organ is supposed to function, and they seek to return that organ to its normal state of function. There are lungs in every body, and we all need to breathe. Doctors seek to help, by sharing the skills and talents they have acquired over the years. They see the truth, which is the perfection behind the disease. They focus on this truth, so that they can help anyone. They see beyond the individual personalities, and they love the process of healing, of helping someone return to a state of health.

Many people who have a love of animals become veterinarians. Veterinarians share that same love of healing, but I think they also have such compassion for animals because animals are so innocent, and often so helpless. It's easy to love an animal, because animals practice unconditional love. Animals love us just because. They are forgiving by nature. They are trusting. They thrive on affection and return it in abundance.

> *"Only the intelligence of love and compassion can solve all problems of life."*
>
> *- Krishnamurti*

Teachers share the knowledge they have acquired with much patience. They see the benefits that come with education and they are happy to share their love of the process. Many teachers choose to teach children because of a love for children. Young children exude love and enthusiasm. They still haven't found any need or desire to be anyone other than who they really are. There is no pretense.

It's easy to love a baby. Babies are untouched by the world. There is no ego, no behavior for us to judge. As time goes on and people age, and the pressures and negativities of life start to challenge us, we have to remember to love. We have to remember the seeds of love we were when we were so young and innocent. When we have issues with another person we can choose to see that love inside of them, to look for that love they were born with that might be covered up at the moment.

If Bhakti Yoga resonates with you, you are likely a people person. You will be happiest in a career where you come into contact with people on a regular basis. You can practice Bhakti no matter what you are doing, or who you are with. You can share a smile, show appreciation and gratitude, take the time to really look in someone's eyes and see who they are. This is bhakti in practice.

The bhakta understands that we are all one, that we are all a part of the whole while at the same time being individual expressions of that whole. It's like God is the sun, are we are each rays of sunlight. We can be far from the sun, but we are never separate from it. When we want to warm our hearts, we only need to move closer to the sun. No ray of sunlight is any less important than any other. We each have our place, and we each have our purpose.

Another analogy that comes up in spiritual texts is that God is the ocean, and we are each individual waves in that ocean. We express ourselves individually, and we merge back into the ocean. While we are the wave, we are still the ocean at the same time. The ocean is made up of many, many waves, and no two are alike. Each is beautiful; each has purpose.

"One drop of the sea cannot claim to come from one river, and another drop of the sea from another river; the sea is a single consistent whole. In the same way all beings are one; there is no being that does not come from the soul, and is not part of the soul."

—*Chandogya Upanishad*

"I am a Bhakta and my purpose is to love."

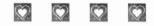

KARMA YOGA
The Path of Work

KARMA YOGA
The Path of Work

"Make your work to be in keeping with your purpose."

– Leonardo da Vinci

WORK AND ACTIVITY

The Sanskrit word "karma" comes from the root "kri" which means "to do." Like many Sanskrit words, karma has several layers of meaning. Karma embodies the definitions of work, activity, or action. There is a law of karma, also quite commonly known as the law of cause and effect, which says that karma is not just our actions, but also the results of our actions.

Any thought, word, or deed, is considered an action. An action will cause an effect, and that effect will then cause whatever comes next. Thus, we have a "law," a predictable sequence of events. Cause leads to effect leads to cause, etc.

Someone on the path of Karma Yoga is known as a Karma Yogi. If you find that you are drawn to this path, then you will find your purpose, your dharma, through the work that you do, the service that you give. You learn from, and express yourself with your actions, and the world benefits.

> *"Freedom is a state of mind – not freedom from something."*
>
> *– Krishnamurti*

The goal of all of the yogas is freedom. And the goal of Karma Yoga is freedom from the bondage of cause and effect. We get caught up in habits, we have certain expectations and we tend to go about our activities on autopilot. These habits create the same outcomes for us, and we wonder why things aren't any different. We feel trapped by our karma, and don't know how to break from it. Yet, we do not have to be bound by the karmic cycles in life. Karma Yoga shows us how, through work and activity, we can be free. Karma Yoga could be called the science of work. It shows us how to work smarter, rather than harder. The Buddha said: *"Do good and be good, and this will take you to freedom, and to whatever truth there is."*

Everything we do is karma. We can't help but think, breathe, act. This is what makes Karma Yoga so easy to practice. We don't have to read or study or worship, we don't have to go anywhere. Sitting is karma, and walking is karma. Karma is our everyday small actions, and overall it is the accumulation of all the actions we have ever taken in our lives. How we live our lives now helps to determine how we will live our lives in the future. The more we understand this the more we see how much power we really have.

Every choice we make is the cause for some effect. We need to make good choices, consciously, keeping in mind that our free will is creating our future.

SELFLESSNESS

For most of us in the west, when we hear the word "work" we think of "job" or "occupation" or "career." It's what we do for a living. Since karma is everything we do, the job we have is a part of the work we do, but that is far from all of it. Karma Yoga shows us that it is not just what we do, but how and why we do it.

When we work a job merely for the paycheck, for the money we receive, that is about all we get out of it. We probably don't look forward to getting up in the morning and dragging ourselves off to work, and we just hang on until payday when we can justify our actions. This doesn't feel good. But, what if we began to see this particular job as a service that we were performing? We can shift our thinking from being selfish, just working for the money, to being selfless, working to serve others. No matter what job you have, there is a reason for it, and when you work to the best of your ability, knowing that this work you are doing is benefiting other people in some way, then work becomes more meaningful. It feels good. We start to feel free.

Yes, we deserve compensation for our efforts. But when we work selflessly we find the compensation to be so much more than money and material gains. Work gives us opportunities to learn and grow by serving. We learn about ourselves and about the people around us. We learn from our experiences, and we become better people, and make better choices. Learning and growing in wisdom is one of the best things that we can do to help the world. Unselfishness leads to expansion, it brings us closer to our goal of freedom. Selfish actions are limiting, and take us further away from freedom. To work selflessly means we have no agenda. Karma Yoga shows us the benefits of work for the sake of work, of helping others. This is selfless service. We realize that when we are helping others, we are also helping ourselves. The attitude must be: "How can I help?" Not: "What's in it for me?" or "You owe me one."

> *"Does a flower, full of beauty, light and loveliness say, 'I am giving, helping, serving?' It is! And because it is not trying to do anything it covers the earth."*
>
> *— Krishnamurti*

The world itself, that we have created, with all the worldly things in it, is by default selfish. There is ownership, and possession. We have property lines, borders, and boundaries. We identify with our job, our house, and our family. And everything we use comes with a price tag attached. There is a kind of agreed-upon value for whatever it is that is available for us to buy. This is the world we live in. But the scriptures, in essence, say that we are "in this world but not of it." We live in the world, but we are not defined by the world.

Someone might say: "I am a native Californian. I am a wife. I am a mother. I am a writer. I am a homeowner." But is that true? These are descriptions, but they are not definitions of who a person really is. Who we are is pure spirit. We are so much more than what we drive, what we wear, where we live, and with whom we socialize. We are creative, limitless, powerful, intelligent, beautiful, and then some! Understanding this is giving up that "self" with a little s and embracing the "Self" with a big S. When we see that each of us is that Self, that individual expression of God, and we are all connected, and here to help each other learn and grow, then all of our actions, all of our karma, will be unselfish. God is selfless, and this is our true nature. This is what Pierre Teilhard de Chardin, a Jesuit priest, meant when he wrote in 1955: "*We are not human beings having a spiritual experience; we are spiritual beings having a human experience.*"

Selfishness brings us misery. It doesn't matter whether we sit on a throne or a stone, whether we live in a palace or a hut, selfishness is a state of mind. It is a matter of: Are we "worldly," attached to the "things" of this world, or are we "Godly?" We only have to look at our behavior to see how selfish we are behaving. We must ask ourselves: What is the priority? Where is our attention?

NON-ATTACHMENT

Karma Yoga teaches us to work, but to give up all attachment to the work itself. That means perform the task, but don't expect anything in return. I learned a phrase when I was sixteen and in my very first self-help type of workshop that has resonated with me all of these years: *"Unfulfilled expectations cause upset."* It's true. If we have an expectation, and it doesn't come to fruition, then we become disappointed. It is better not to have any expectation, to give up an attachment to any kind of outcome, and just be grateful for the experience itself, rather than counting on a particular result. Upset, or misery, comes from the attachment to the things of the world, not from the work itself.

The title that we have in any particular job is something that we could become attached to as well. The president of a corporation wields a certain amount of status and power. But we need to remember that the status and power come with the position. Whoever holds that title is that one who has the responsibility during that time. But the title can go away at any time. So when we lose a title, what have we really lost? Changing jobs is like changing hats. We play our roles, and then go on to the next. All the while, we are the same person. Our real power doesn't come from any particular title or job, our real power comes from within.

What do we expect when we work? We often expect praise, gratitude, reward, enjoyment, or some sort of result. But sometimes those things just don't come. And then how do we feel? Let down, disappointed, used. Maybe even angry, or hurt. This doesn't feel good. But then the feeling passes. Sooner or later you feel fine again. All of these feelings, the pain, the pleasures, are temporary, they are fleeting. So are the things of the world. The job, paycheck, the wealth, the poverty, the car, the house, even the people in our lives – they are here for a while, and then they're not. They exist in a certain place and time and then they move on. There is no use in calling anything "mine." Any sense of possession carries with it selfishness, and selfishness brings on misery. We become slaves to our possessions, they tie us down, burden us, restricting our freedom.

Let's look at a car for example. The car has a Mercedes emblem on it. It has a license plate holder with the dealership information displayed. A person with a job as a sales representative drives the car. The sales rep works for a company that financed the car through a bank. The car is parked in a public parking lot. Whose car is it? At any given time you could make an argument for any of the parties involved.

It doesn't matter what you have. What is important is how you feel about what you have. One might say: "This is *my* car, I worked hard to pay for this car, I picked out this car, I drive this car." If you feel attached to that car, and the car is stolen, or wrecked, then you become upset. You feel a loss. You worry. You feel bad. The misery comes from the attachment to the car. If, on the other hand, you are not attached to the car, but instead look at the car for what it is – a temporary object that provides transportation – then whatever happens to that car does not cause you misery. You might even feel gratitude for the time you had the car. By the same token, when we win a new car in a contest, we maintain our peace of mind, and do not get overly excited. We understand that a car, or any particular object, is not what brings us happiness. There is a kind of humility that comes with knowing that God is present at all times, in success and failure, in losses and gains. There is a calm confidence in knowing that everything is just fine, that whatever needs to happen will happen.

"How many cares one loses when one decides not to be something but to be someone."

–Coco Chanel

Karma Yoga shows us that it is best to enjoy the beauty of the world, but not to identify with it. Everything belongs to God. And if we are a part of God, then everything belongs to us anyway! We are just here to use it, to enjoy it, to appreciate it. It's like when we go to the theatre to see a play. We are given a ticket, and taken to a seat. You might say: "This is my seat." And for that particular performance, yes, it is your seat. No one else sits in it but you. But then the audience files out and the next show starts and someone else has that seat. It is theirs. We take the seat, and then we give it back to God. It is ours for a moment, and then it is not. We can enjoy it, and appreciate it, while we have it, but not be attached to it. We can't exactly carry it out of the theatre with us!

CHANGE

And that's the same way it goes with all the things of the world. As they say: "You can't take it with you." There's no point in being attached to anything we have because we end up leaving it all behind when we exit anyway. Even something as big and seemingly permanent as a house can't really belong to us. The land was there long before the house was. Someone or some committee decided where lines were going to be drawn and houses built. Someone lived in the house before you, and someone will live there after you. You may be making payments to a bank that holds the title. The house really isn't something you own, it's a place for you to live. If you understand this and can keep it in perspective, then you won't be upset when you move, or the house burns down, or every time the plumbing breaks down or repairs are necessary.

In May of 2010 Norman, Oklahoma was hit with a huge tornado. My stepsister, Debby Kaspari and her husband, Mike, were right in its path. Their home, garden, barn, trees, cars, everything was literally blown apart and away in a matter of seconds. Thankfully, Debby and Mike and their cat Gizmo were tucked away safely in their storm shelter and they walked away without a scratch.

What happens when everything that represents stability and comfort in life is suddenly and violently ripped away in a matter of minutes? You cling to what you know is really important, your relationships, your strength, your resilience. Debby is an artist, an amazing artist (she created the peacock on the cover of this book), and she keeps a blog. She was able to chronicle her experience and share some of the miracles that happened along the way. A treasured banjo was rescued, her precious sketchbooks, representing years of work, were found. And amidst all the chaos and destruction, love shone through! As Debby writes: *"Disaster brings out the greatness of a community. After the shock came an outpouring of support; there were heroes all around us. I've now seen angels with chainsaws, driving forklifts, filling out paperwork and bearing lasagna casseroles."*

This support is Karma Yoga in action. Volunteers, friends, and neighbors, all came together for the good of the whole. No selfishness, just help, just work. Each contributed what they could, in whatever way they were able. There was so much compassion exhibited because they could each relate to what this couple was going through. Had the tornado come one block further or one street over, it easily could have been another house that was devastated. Things can be replaced. When something like this happens, we see and feel the real ties that bind us, we know what is really important. We see this over and over again when disaster strikes. As horrible as things look on the outside, the love, the spirit, can never be destroyed. Things are temporary, emotions are fleeting, conditions change for better or worse, but love is everlasting, and God is always present.

IMPERMANENCE

The sand mandala is a Tibetan Buddhist tradition involving the creation and also destruction of mandalas made from colored sand. I had the pleasure of watching this all happen during a trip to India. In the ritual, a group of monks create an elaborate and very intricately designed piece of art in the shape of a circle using colored sand. The artwork holds much symbolism, and is geometrically laid out in detail. It can take days, and even weeks to build the mandala, as each monk uses special tools to pour the sand in just the right way to create the design.

They start from the center and move outward, and usually work in shifts around the clock. They work quietly, with much concentration and attention. It is quite intense, and absolutely beautiful with all of the colors.

Once the mandala is complete it is surrounded by candles and there is often chanting performed around it. This is when we stand in awe at the beauty of this mandala, when we take in its beauty, and express gratitude for having witnessed it. And then, in a very ritualistic ceremony, one monk stands and sweeps the mandala away. All of the sand blends together. The design is gone, the colors merge to become a kind of tan and gray, and we are left with a pile of sand. The destruction of the mandala is done as a metaphor of the impermanence of life. It is a reminder to us to appreciate and be grateful for what is before us while it is there. It is a symbol of the Buddhist doctrinal belief in the transitory nature of material life.

The sand is swept up and placed in an urn. Half of the sand is distributed to those watching the closing ceremony. I have a little vial of sand that I kept to remember this experience. The other half is carried to a nearby body of water, where it is deposited. The waters then carry the healing blessing to the ocean, and from there it spreads throughout the world for planetary healing. So although the mandala, in all its glory, is no longer physically present, it still serves a very important purpose. Nothing is ever wasted.

The repercussions are felt far and wide. The gifts continue to flow. And for that we can be grateful. The lesson in impermanence is a lesson in unattachment. Enjoy what comes, and then give it back.

RELATIONSHIPS

As much as we love the people in our lives, we must remain unattached to them as well. We don't possess them; we don't own them. We are connected to each other, but we are not bound to each other. Relationships change. Even our own children, who grow inside of us, are not "ours." Kahlil Gibran's poem "On Children" expresses this so beautifully:

Your children are not your children.
They are the sons and daughters of Life's longing
for itself.
They come through you but not from you,
And though they are with you yet they belong not to you.

You may give them your love but not your thoughts,
For they have their own thoughts.
You may house their bodies but not their souls,
For their souls dwell in the house of tomorrow,
which you cannot visit, not even in your dreams.
You may strive to be like them,
but seek not to make them like you.
For life goes not backward nor tarries with yesterday.

You are the bows from which your children
as living arrows are sent forth.

The archer sees the mark upon the path of the infinite,
and He bends you with His might
that His arrows may go swift and far.
Let your bending in the archer's hand be for gladness;
For even as He loves the arrow that flies,
so He loves also the bow that is stable.

Our first relationship is with our self. We come into this world with a body, and we claim that this is our body. And for the time that we are on this earth, living this human existence, the body is here to serve us. The body is a tool for us to use in order to serve others, to do the work that we need to do. As the years go on, the body changes, and these changes might even remind us that our time in this particular body is limited. So it is important to take care of the body, so that it can support us optimally in our goals. Keep it clean. Eat good foods so that it gets the nutrients it needs to stay healthy. Exercise to keep the bones and muscles functioning the way they need to. The longer we live, the healthier we are, the more chance we have to serve others, to learn and grow, and to gain wisdom.

It is also important to recognize that because our time is limited, it is foolish to waste it. The work we do is important for ourselves and for all of humanity. Every moment counts. That is not to say that our lives need to be filled with being busy. Quite the contrary! We need balance in our lives. Time spent doing "nothing" can actually be very productive when we are meditating, contemplating, re-charging our batteries, praying, experiencing our connection with God. Meditation and action are of equally significant to us. Meditation teaches us to have that peace of mind amidst our activity. Karma Yoga calls us to action, to be involved, to participate in the world and its events, rather than to seclude ourselves. But when this activity is focused and grounded then we are more productive and our time is used more effectively and efficiently. We are at peace when we work, even when the work is difficult. We are able to make better decisions. Our activity can be a spiritual activity.

GIVING UP ATTACHMENT

Karma Yoga explains that there are two ways that we can shed ourselves of attachments. The first is to make a conscious effort mentally to see things as they are, not as we think they should be, not as we wish they could be. This takes a shift in thinking, and it requires practice. What we are really doing is detaching from the outcome of any given circumstance. We are living in the present moment, not wanting or needing to change anything. It's about giving up our human need for control, letting go of that thought that we know better, or that we have all the answers. When we give up attachment we are aware that change happens, and we accept it. We don't try to manipulate it.

The second way to give up attachment is to do whatever it is that we do, for God. Rather than working for a paycheck, work for God. Work to serve God. Work to show love for God. This is Karma Yoga. When there is no outside motive, not the motive of pay or praise, then the work we do is selfless. We can work very hard, for long hours, and the time just flies by. We don't feel tired, we feel energized. We love what we do, because it makes us feel good. What was a job becomes a joy. The Bhagavad Gita says:

> *Whatever your action,*
> *Food or worship;*
> *Whatever the gift*
> *That you give to another;*
> *Whatever you vow*
> *To the work of the spirit...*
> *Lay these also*
> *As offerings before Me.*

In Karma Yoga, work is a form of worship. We do the best that we can, we challenge ourselves to always do better, because we want to learn and grow, we want to see ourselves progress. We want to express ourselves, and our love, and we do that through our work. Our work is our duty, and it is also our great opportunity, it is a gift. Life is holy, and work can be holy, too.

GIVING

When we practice Karma Yoga, we intentionally seek to help others. And we know that by helping others, we are also helping ourselves. We are all connected, so we can't really help anyone but ourselves. Everyone we see is an extension of ourselves. When we give to others, we give to ourselves. The goal of Karma Yoga is self-realization. When we know ourselves, we know the world.

Many people explain karma as "what goes around, comes around." By that they mean that whatever we put out into the universe eventually comes back to us. We don't have to keep score, the universe takes care of all that. But there does seem to be some balance at play here. When we are kind, then that kindness is generally returned. It might not be immediately, but when we are in need of that favor, or that gentle word, then it tends to come to us, maybe from somewhere we never would have expected.

"Give with faith, and never without faith. Give with dignity. Give with humility. Give with joy. And give with understanding of the effects of your gift."

—Taittiriya Upanishad

Giving can be a part of our culture, a way of life. Blake Mycoskie is the founder of TOMS, an innovative "One for One" company. It all started when Blake was traveling in Argentina, and he befriended children who had no shoes to protect their feet. Wanting to help these kids, he went back to the U.S. and created TOMS, a company that matches every pair of shoes purchased with a pair of new shoes given to a child in need. Blake says: "Giving is what fuels us. Giving is our future." The name TOMS comes from his idea that someone buys a pair of shoes today, so they can give a pair tomorrow, so they are shoes for tomorrow, or TOMS for short, to fit on the label. Blake Mycoskie is an example of a Karma Yogi. He is living his dharma, working both hard and creatively. He provides jobs, and he helps the world. Now TOMS has branched out and is doing the same "One for One" giving with eyewear as well as shoes.

The only way to really give is to give without expectation. That is, to give without expectation of getting anything in return. Don't expect praise, or even gratitude. Don't expect any reward. Give for the sake of giving. Help for the sake of helping. Buddhism explains that desire, whether it is the desire for money, or love, or credit, whatever it is, leads to suffering. And this is because our desires can never truly be fulfilled. They always leave us wanting for more. One desire is then replaced with another. It's never enough. Have no desires, have no expectations, and then we will have no suffering. We need to give up our attachment to desire so that we can be happy. Swami Vivekananda said: *"Give up all fruits of work; do good for its own sake, then alone will come perfect non-attachment. The bonds of the heart will thus break, and we shall realize perfect freedom. This freedom is indeed the goal of Karma Yoga."*

SERVICE

Karma Yoga is not about charity, or philanthropy, it is about service. There is a big difference here. Of course philanthropy is a good thing. The difference is that when we are mindfully and intentionally being of service, we understand that we are privileged to have the opportunity to help others. We know that when we are doing good, and helping others, we are becoming closer to God. And then there is a realization that all these others that you are helping are really an extension of yourself. You really can't help anyone but yourself. There is a spiritual maturity that is a part of service. Karma Yoga explains that all the work we do, is really work for ourselves, on ourselves.

> *"All growth depends upon activity. There is no development physically or intellectually without effort, and effort means work. Work is not a curse; it is the prerogative of intelligence... the measure of civilization."*

> *– Calvin Coolidge*

We can do what needs to be done because it is simply good to do good. In this way, we can transform the world. The Buddha said: *"Do good and be good, and this will take you to freedom and whatever truth there is."* Every good deed counts, every good thought, every kind gesture. Doing good can be a habit, a part of our nature, our first instinct. This is how we get to a state of unselfishness. We can get beyond motives of fame or money or prestige and even the motive of enlightenment, and work for the sake of work itself.

With each of the four Yogas, the secret to its effectiveness is the practice. We can read about it, we can understand what we have to do, but we truly understand our purpose when we put the philosophy into practice. With Karma Yoga, there's really no excuse not to practice, because there is always work to do. Work is never ending. There is continually something that needs to be done. Do the work that needs to be done, knowing that this is a part of your dharma.

> *"What, then, is your duty? What the day demands."*
>
> *– Johann Wolfgang von Goethe*

THE GHOST STORY

Swami Vivekananda, known for his teachings on Vedanta, would tell the story of a poor man who had heard that if he could get a ghost to work for him, he would have all of his heart's desires. He searched for someone who could give him the magic to conjure up such a ghost. He finally came upon a sage, and begged him so much that the sage eventually broke down, and against his better judgment gave the man a magic word to repeat that would summon such a ghost. The sage told the man that this ghost would do whatever the man told him to, but that he must be kept continually busy. If the man failed to give him work, the ghost would kill him. The man felt confident that he could keep the ghost occupied, and so he used the magic word and the ghost presented himself. The ghost issued the man the same warning, saying: "The moment you fail to give me work I will kill you."

The man began shouting orders out to the ghost, and demanded a palace. With the snap of a finger the ghost produced the palace: "Done," he said. "Give me money!" said the man, and in no time at all, the ghost presented him with piles of it. Then the man told the ghost to replace the forest with a city, and that, too, the ghost did in an instant. "What else?" the ghost insisted. "If you have no further employment for me then I will eat you." The man grew frightened, he couldn't think of anything more for the ghost to do. He could see that the ghost could do everything so quickly that it was impossible to keep him occupied.

The man ran as fast as he could back to the sage and begged for the sage to save his life. The sage agreed to help him, and told the man to pick up his dog with a curly tail: "Give this dog to the ghost, and tell him to straighten out the dog's tail." The man did as the sage told him, and gave the dog to the ghost: "Straighten out this tail for me," he said. The ghost took the dog, and slowly and deliberately straightened out the tail. But once he let the tail go, it curled right up again. The ghost again straightened out the tail, only to have it curl up once more. He tried again and again, over several days. Finally exhausted, the ghost said to the man: "I am an old ghost, and I have never had a task give me so many problems. I will make a deal with you. Let me go, and you can keep all the treasures and I will not harm you." The man was relieved and happily accepted the offer.

Karma Yoga tells us that the world is like a dog's curly tail. We've been striving for hundreds of years to straighten it out, but it always goes back to curly. This is its nature. We must come to the understanding that this is the way it is. We have to work without attachment, and not be obsessed with making things the way we think they should be.

WHAT NEEDS TO BE DONE

Mothers understand that work is never ending. No sooner do the dishes get done than they get dirtied again. The laundry is clean, folded and put away, and then the basket is full again. The kids get dropped off, and then they need to be picked up. We can't ignore these things or there would be total chaos in the house. We do what needs to be done. We can't expect the house to stay spotless because it just doesn't. If anyone has this expectation then that expectation causes turmoil in the household, and all kinds of nervousness and anxiety manifests. Remember: *"Unfulfilled expectations cause upset."* So, let it go. Or as it is often said: *"Let Go and Let God."*

The world will do what it does, no matter what we do. So the best we can do is to release our attachment to the outcome and just do our work. We have to be calm and make good choices and put in our best efforts doing what needs to be done. We can't get discouraged or disappointed when things don't turn out the way we want them to. Things turn out the way they are supposed to.

It is a privilege for each of us to work, to do our part for the world. The world is not beholding to any of us. Instead know that it is an honor, a gift that we are given to do our part to help the world. In helping the world, we are helping ourselves. The world does not need our help; there is an organizing power to the universe and it functions just fine without us. We are given this opportunity to participate, and it is to our benefit to accept it.

> *"No matter how insignificant the thing you have to do, do it as well as you can, give it as much of our care and attention as you would give to the thing you regard as most important."*

> *– Mahatma Gandhi*

We have to understand that we can't change the world; we can't make it the perfect place we would like it to be. It already is perfect in its imperfections! But we can change ourselves. We can learn to be more wise, and compassionate. We can practice Karma Yoga and do some good. There is a Buddhist saying that when you are stepping on rocks, ask yourself: Is it better to cover the earth in leather, or to put on a pair of shoes?

OUR THOUGHTS, WORDS AND DEEDS

"The main purpose of life is to live rightly, think rightly, act rightly. The soul must languish when we give all our thought to the body."

– *Mahatma Gandhi*

There is a saying that actions speak louder than words. And this is true. When we say one thing and do another thing, then we are contradicting ourselves, and the action is what will win out. Yet our words carry weight. Karma Yoga tells us that speech is an action. We need to be mindful of the words that we speak, because they have an impact on us, and on the world. By the same token, we need to be mindful of what we think. Swami Vivekananda says that wondering is the first step in the acquisition of wisdom. There is a relationship between thought and word. We think, then speak, then someone hears us, and thinks about what we are saying. Our words are formed by our thoughts. Our words are powerful because they can elicit an emotional response.

When a child is hurt, imagine the effect a few kind words, gently spoken, can have. Tears dry up, and she is comforted, and calm. Think about how words can get a crowd riled up at a political rally. Or how the broadcast of a tragedy can cause sadness and despair in people all over the world. Being able to consciously use our words to heal, to thoughtfully and intentionally help rather than hurt, is a part of Karma Yoga. Speak the truth. Do what you say you are going to do. Be humble. Do not gossip or spread rumors. Always do your best. And keep the company of others who have such integrity as well.

Having integrity is our personal responsibility, and I believe it is also the responsibility of the media as well. The media projects vibrations out into the universe with every story that it reports. There is a huge influence on the public's emotions and perceptions. Actions cause reactions, which in turn cause actions. Causes produce effects. When a thought, word, or action causes an effect, this is karma. We need to be careful about what we put out into the world. We can describe this as care-full rather than care-less, doing what needs to be done mindfully, rather than going after sensationalism or exploitation for the sake of ratings.

"In nature, action and reaction are continuous. Everything is connected to everything else. No one part, nothing, is isolated. Everything is linked, and interdependent. Everywhere everything is connected to everything else. Each question receives the correct answer."

– Swami Prajnanpad

In the media we see tragedy, and we see triumph. We have seen the devastation that happens on the other side of the world when a natural disaster occurs. And we see how that devastation affects each of us. We are all connected, and we reach out to others to participate in their healing and recovery. With bad comes good, and with good comes bad. They are two sides of the same coin and the nature of this world. We can't get too attached to the misery, just as we can't get too attached to elation. They are both fleeting in the long run. The Olympics is a time when the world comes together in celebration. It is glorious and inspiring. It is wonderful to enjoy the moments while they occur. And yet, those moments come to an end. Life goes on, and work continues, and we must carry on. We can't be attached to the past and we can't have any expectations for the future. The best we can do is to live in the present moment and mindfully do the work we need to do. In this way we spiritualize our lives. The Bhagavad Gita says: *"Thus you will free yourself from both the good and the evil effects of your actions."*

Oprah Winfrey is a Karma Yogi. She has chosen to use the media as a platform to help people to learn and grow. During the 25 years that she hosted and produced her talk show she covered issues that were of deep concern to people all over the world. And she was able to do so in such a way that we were given tools to make things better, for ourselves and for others. And now she has an even larger platform through which to express her dharma. Her message of "Live Your Best Life" resonates with so many of us. Oprah truly is making a difference in this world every single day.

BALANCE AND IMBALANCE

Overall there is balance in the world, but it's the current state of imbalance that leads us to strive for change, that compels us forward, that helps us to grow. If everything were hunky-dory all the time we would not be as motivated to work. It's in the wanting things to be better, the struggle to achieve, that fires our imagination and leads us to tap into our creativity. We are a part of nature's plan. We are here with our human nature to work and get things done. We just have to do our jobs without attachment to the outcome knowing that God, or Nature, knows much more than we do.

We can practice self-control by watching what we take in to our minds, and what comes out of our mouths. The more we practice, the less influence that outside sources have on our peace of mind. We know that the world is not always as it appears to be, and that there is indeed harmony, and purpose to everything and everyone. Karma Yoga teaches that through our every day actions we can become free.

THE SCIENCE OF WORK

Karma Yoga can be looked at as the science of work. There is a natural three-step process we experience that leads us to freedom. We do all of this through practice.

1. Selfless Activity. Give up attachment to any reward, to any expectation of what will come of your labor, and simply work for the sake of work. Do what needs to be done. Take the necessary steps.

2. Work As Worship. Now, instead of working just for work, work for God. See work as an offering of love. Do your best. Put yourself into your work. You'll find that you start to enjoy your work, that it's not a chore but a pleasure. Work can be a meditation, where you lose track of time. Time simply flies by without your awareness.

3. God As Worker. Finally, we understand that there is a Oneness in the world and in our activity. God is working through us, for us, for each of us and for all of us because we are all part of the same Whole. Work is now effortless, and also meaningful. We are filled with gratitude.

"It is in the very heart of our activity that we search for our goal."

– Rabindranath Tagore

EXPRESSIONS OF KARMA YOGA

The beauty of Karma Yoga is that is can be practiced and expressed in any occupation, in any activity, at any time. If Karma Yoga resonates with you, then you might consider how you can incorporate the practice into all aspects of your life. It's the mindset that work is not a chore, but a gift. It's looking for work, and welcoming it rather than avoiding it. It's using every opportunity that presents itself to do some good.

"I believe in hard work. It keeps the wrinkles out of the mind and the spirit."

– Helena Rubinstein

Karma Yogis can be found in professions that provide a service. Traditionally this would include police officers and fire fighters, where helping people is a part of the job description. These people are often known as "public servants." People who hold public office might also fit in this category, at least the ones who have deliberately sought office to make a difference in the world and change things for the better.

Karma Yoga is prevalent in the hotel industry, or the restaurant business, both of which would be classified under "hospitality." Athletes, who are so committed to the work of training and practicing and being part of a team, are also often Karma Yogis. To sacrifice personal hours, get up so early in the morning to train, whatever the weather, takes dedication. To continue on through injuries shows a love for the work.

When you need to get something done, it's great to have a Karma Yogi on your team. This is a person who perseveres, who doesn't give up. This is a person who rises to the occasion and gets the job done.

> *"There is no greater satisfaction for a just and well-meaning person than the knowledge that he has devoted his best energies to the service of the good cause."*
>
> – *Albert Einstein*

"I am a Karma Yogi and my purpose is to serve."

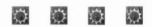

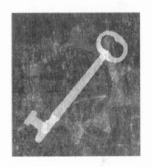

JNANA YOGA
The Path of Knowledge

JNANA YOGA
The Path of Knowledge

"Knowledge is the annihilation of the separation between me and the other."

– Swami Prajnanpad

KNOWLEDGE AND WISDOM

The goal of Jnana Yoga, as it is with the other yogas, is freedom. And the way freedom is attained in Jnana Yoga is with knowledge, knowledge of the self, and of our Oneness with God and all that is. The Jnana Yogi uses the powers of the intellect to achieve mastery over the mind, mastery over the many distractions and emotions in the world that would have us believe that we are separate.

If you are drawn to the path of Jnana Yoga, then you will find your dharma is through knowledge and study. You are a thinker, and you can figure things out by using your mind, taking in various theories and explanations. You can process concepts that might be considered complicated or difficult and come to your own conclusions. You piece together parts of the puzzle to come to a deeper understanding of the world and your place in it.

Everything we see, touch, smell, hear, or taste – this is a part of conditional reality. These things exist under certain conditions, and they appear to be separate from our selves. Our senses keep us connected to our human existence. The house we live in, the chair we sit in, the people we talk with – all of this appears to be distinct and individual. And yet this is our conditional reality. All of these "things" of life are temporary. They have a lifespan in time and space. They are subject to change. They are imperfect. On the other hand, all that is eternal, perfect and unchanging is defined as ultimate reality. This is the unseen, and this is what is truly real. This is God, or Brahman, and this is the reality that encompasses everything, including our selves.

Steve Jobs is an example of someone who lived his life as a Jnana Yogi. He was an inventor and an entrepreneur who always thought ahead, anticipating and dreaming up possibilities that he could put into form and function. Steve, along with some of his close friends, founded Apple, the company responsible for one of the first commercially successful lines of personal computers. Steve has been quoted as saying: "You can't just ask customers what they want and then try to give that to them. By the time you get it built, they'll want something new."

In 1985 Steve lost a power struggle with the Apple board of directors and he left the company. Although this was devastating for him at the time, he would later say that it was one of the best things that happened to him, because of how much he learned and was able to grow from the experience. This is a great lesson for us in non-attachment. He acquired the computer graphics division of Lucasfilm Ltd, which was spun off as Pixar Animation Studios, another highly innovative and creative company that changed the world of animation. Later Steve returned to Apple and served as CEO, leading the advent of the iPod, iPhone and iPad. As successful as he was, Steve felt it was most important that he make some contribution to the world. He said in a 1993 Wall Street Journal interview: "Being the richest man in the cemetery doesn't matter to me. Going to bed at night saying we've done something wonderful, that's what matters to me."

When Steve died in 2011 it was amazing to see all the tributes posted online. He touched so many people with his amazing inventions, and also by the way he lived his own life.

MAYA

In Jnana Yoga, the philosophy is that there is a "veil of illusion" that keeps us from knowing our true nature and the nature of the world around us. That illusion is called "maya." When we start to tear a hole in that veil, we see more clearly, we see things as they are. The more we learn and grow, the larger the hole becomes, and the easier it is for us to see and know what is real. Mental discipline allows us to break through maya, as we train our mind using both a negative and positive approach in our discernment:

1. First look at what it not really real. "Neti, neti" means "not this, not this." We first need to look at what is unreal, and understand that anything impermanent (the "stuff" of the world – including possessions) is not real. It comes, and it goes. Where does it come from, where does it go to? God. For a moment in time it looks like it's real, but it is functioning as an expression of the divine, it is not the whole.

2. Then we look at what *is* real, what is infinite, unbounded, and limitless. The Upanishads say that God is "beyond the reach of

speech and mind." God is all inclusive, all-encompassing, all knowing. This is the positive part – recognizing everything around us as divine because it is a part of the One.

"Just as a man who steps upon a serpent shutters in fear but then looks down and notices it is only a rope, so it was that one day I realized that what I was calling "I" cannot be found, and all fear and anxiety vanished with my mistake."

– The Buddha

The idea is to replace ignorance with knowledge. Jnana Yoga gives a few tools with which we can do just that.

DISCRIMINATION

Discrimination is differentiating between the real and the unreal at any given time. It is seeing the real behind the unreal. Life is like one big movie. When we're sitting in the movie theater and the movie comes on, we know that it is just a show. But we get caught up in the story. We feel the emotions; we get taken for a ride. But when we think about it, we know that these are actors playing out a scene and, that these are characters and not "real" people. And what they are doing isn't "really" happening. Then if we take it a step further, we know also that this is just a picture on a screen. The actors are not in front of us. The picture isn't real; it's light and color projected onto a screen. Discrimination is being able to recognize that screen behind the action. It's an understanding that despite how everything appears, there is that ultimate reality at work.

Real vs. Unreal

When we look at life as a movie, then we can see that we are writing the script with our actions. Every decision we make, every word we speak, becomes a part of our story. And when we understand that this is the same for every person on this planet, and that we share this experience, then we develop empathy and compassion. We see ourselves in other people, like a reflection in the mirror. We find that there is no need to gossip or argue, because we know how self-damaging that can be. We learn to analyze ourselves and look at our own actions rather than analyzing another person, or placing blame. Our dialogue becomes one of "how can I help" and "what is my role here."

When we feel isolated and alone, when we see ourselves as separate. We then shut ourselves off from the love that is in us and around us at all times. The way we find peace is to remember who we are. We can see ourselves in everything and everyone. We can spiritualize all things, everything is a gift; everything is a reflection of the self.

When we recognize our oneness, we stop feeling alone and separate, and stop depriving ourselves of love. We stop living in fear and anxiety, and allow ourselves to live in love, knowing that we are not alone. We seek peace. Jnana Yoga teaches us that there is no peace in isolation, because we are all connected. So we reach out to others. Then we see that because we are all connected, and because divinity is indivisible, that humans are indeed divine creatures. The knowledge of who we are is evident in our words and actions. We treat each other with care and respect.

Once we understand the difference between what is real and unreal, then it is easier for us to determine just what it is we want. "What do I want?" becomes a much bigger question. Our priorities change, and we understand what is really important to us, and in life in general. What do you *really* want?

> "We do not progress from error to truth, but from truth to truth. Thus we must see that none can be blamed for what they are doing, because they are, at this time, doing the best they can. We learn only from experience."

> – Swami Vivekanana

Our mind plays tricks on us, so we must be diligent in our practice to have mastery over the mind. We have to get ourselves into these good habits so that it is natural for us, as it should be, to have mastery over the mind. Jnana Yoga teaches us to wake up and recognize what is real. When we know this, there is no fear, there is no need to argue, and there is no need to fight or gossip. We are all One, so we know that in hurting another, we are really hurting ourselves. Jnana Yoga helps us to achieve patience, and a sympathetic understanding of what others are going through. It teaches us to accept, and not merely tolerate, all people because we know that there really are no differences between us. The differences we perceive are because of our name and form. We have labeled these things because they look different to us. But when the veil of maya is removed, we see clearly that we are all the same, we are all One: free, perfect, infinite and immortal. We see this in others, and we see this in ourselves as well.

With this in mind, I created an online program called The Kindness Movement (www.EverythingKind.com). The idea behind this campaign is that kindness is contagious. By actively demonstrating kindness we are setting a good example, and helping the world to be a kinder, gentler place where we all can feel more comfortable being who we are.

THE KINDNESS MOVEMENT

Ellen DeGeneres inspired the creation of The Kindness Movement. At the end of her show she says: "Be kind to one another." I love that! The Kindness Movement is about putting that simple statement into ACTION. This is a way we can learn how good kindness feels.

There are 7 days in this experience. Each one is meant to intellectually break down the concept of kindness into a formula that we can all use in our lives. When you sign up on the website you will receive a message in your e-mail box every day for 7 days with some ideas to both think about and act upon. I'm printing them here so that you have them as a reference in this book. Take these messages to heart, use them mindfully throughout your day, and see just how being kind affects the people and the space all around you.

DAY 1:

We all know what kindness is NOT. It's not anger, hatred, bullying, intolerance, or violence. We see these things, or hear them, and it makes us feel bad, it causes us pain. Even when we are not the ones being targeted, it does hurt our hearts, because we are all connected. What hurts one of us hurts all of us. Kindness is the anti-dote to all of this. When we are proactive, when we are consciously practicing kindness we can disarm any negativity around. Kindness is powerful, and precious at the same time. We appreciate kindness, we recognize it, and we honor it.

"No act of kindness, no matter how small, is ever wasted."

– Aesop

Today, be ATTENTIVE. Pay attention to the words you use. Pay attention to the messages you are sending verbally and otherwise. Choose to use a calm and gentle tone of voice. Choose to ask, rather than demand. Take note when others are being kind, and express gratitude. See the many ways that kindness is demonstrated to you, and come up with ideas for ways that you can show kindness toward others.

DAY 2:

Living on this planet together is a shared experience. We're not alone in this world. Every action we take has some sort of an effect on everyone else in some way or another.

"True kindness presupposes the faculty of imagining as one's own the sufferings and joy of others."

– André Gide (1869-1951)

Today, be RECEPTIVE. Sometimes the best thing we can do to be kind is to listen. Be open to hearing what someone else is going through. Listen with your heart. Be quiet and let the other person talk. Make eye contact; connect. We can lessen the pain or amplify the joy just by being there for another person.

DAY 3:

Just as there are many different varieties of flowers in the world, many different trees, all beautiful in their own way, there are also many different people here on earth. No two are alike. And yet, our similarities are more relevant than our differences. We breathe the same air; we feel the same emotions.

"Kindness can become its own motive. We are made kind by being kind."

— *Eric Hoffer (1902-1983)*

Today, be ACCEPTING. Being accepting sounds so passive, so easy. And yet, how many times do we judge people? How many times do we impose our own values on people? How often do we try to change people? Being accepting means allowing "what is" to be as it is. It's knowing that we are each here purposely, and purposefully, to make the world a better place, each in our own way. Respect one another, and understand that we each have our own unique gifts and talents to share.

DAY 4:

The Law of Relationship says that we are all connected, and that we are here to help each other learn and grow. We are not here to hurt each other, or hinder each other. When we do so we are only hurting ourselves, whether we realize it or not.

"What do we live for, if it is not to make life less difficult to each other?"

– *George Eliot*

Today, be HELPFUL. Remember the "big picture." When you can lend a hand, help out. There will be times when you need a hand, too. Live in the present, being aware of what needs to be done in the moment. There are opportunities to be kind and helpful all around at any time. And also be mindful of the future. What we do now affects what happens tomorrow. Be a good guest on this planet: bring your own bags to the grocery store, don't use more than you need, and volunteer your time to help others.

DAY 5:

It's always easier to walk into a room full of friends rather than a room full of strangers. We're all connected, so we're more than friends, we're related! When we treat each other as friends we create a warm and comfortable environment where we can all thrive.

"Kind looks, kind words, kind acts, and warm handshakes – these are secondary means of grace when [people] are in trouble and are fighting their unseen battles."

– *John Hall*

Today, be FRIENDLY. Small gestures of kindness can make a big difference in someone's life. We each struggle at some time or another, and by showing a little kindness, encouragement, or support, we can ease the burden for someone. Sometimes a smile is all it takes to bring sunshine into another person's day. We never know what is going on behind the scenes, or behind someone's eyes. Being friendly is a nice way to show kindness.

DAY 6:

In Ayurveda, India's "Science of Life," all foods are classified into six tastes: sweet, sour, salty, bitter, pungent, and astringent. If these words were being used to describe a personality, which person would you most like to encounter? I think the sweet person would be the most popular hands down! Sweetness takes away the bitterness; sweetness is what we like the most, and why we save dessert for last. When we are in love, we call each other honey, sugar, sweetie, cupcake, or muffin – because these are all "sweet" words and sweetness is associated with love and kindness.

"Kindness in ourselves is the honey that blunts the sting of unkindness in another."

– Walter Savage Landor (1775-1864)

Today, be SWEET. And speak sweetly. Do a favor for someone. Offer a sincere compliment. Surprise someone with a sweet note or a little gift. No expectations for anything in return, in fact you may even want to do this anonymously. Just enjoy being sweet, and see how good it makes you feel.

DAY 7:

There can be a shift at any time, including right here and now. It can be a shift in thinking, a shift in attitude, or even a shift in direction of where we are headed into the future. Because we want to live in a kinder, gentler world, we need to practice right where we are. One by one, we will make a difference.

"Kindness is ever the begetter of kindness."

– Sophocles

Today, be GIVING. And also be forgiving. No one is perfect; we all make mistakes. The important thing is to learn from our mistakes, correct them, and behave more kindly and authentically the next opportunity we have. Offer an apology when you mess up. We have to give each other, and ourselves, a break sometimes! Kindness is our nature, so being kind feels good because it is natural. When we are kind, we are being true to ourselves, and to each other. Give of yourself, of your time, talents, and treasures. We each have so much to share that can benefit so many people.

We could sit in the dark, or we could turn on a light. We could live amongst hatred, or we could bring in love. We could live in a nightmare, or we could wake up! We understand these options in our minds, and we need to take the necessary steps to live the lives we want to lead. Intentionally and purposefully, we can one by one reveal the bright shiny world beneath the veil. It starts with each one of us.

> *"When the life of a man, freed from all distractions, finds its unity in the spirit, the knowledge of the infinite comes to him immediately and naturally, like light from a flame."*

> *– Rabindranath Tagore*

Jnana Yoga says that it is our intellect that will get us to the point where we see the divine in all. We must make the choice to learn and grow, to overcome any ignorance and shed the veil of maya. Maya is all around us. It's like a doughnut that looks rich and delicious but that leaves us feeling bloated and undernourished after we've eaten it. Maya is an empty promise, unfulfilling and ultimately disappointing.

In his book "The Tao of Physics" Fritjof Capra says: *"Maya does not mean that the world is an illusion, as is often wrongly stated. The illusion merely lies in our point of view. Maya is the illusion of mistaking our relative perspective for reality, of confusing the map with the territory."* The philosophy behind all of this is that the material world exists, yet it is temporary. When we see it as permanent, then we are mistaken. Material things are measurable, they take place in space and time. What is permanent is the spiritual, which takes place beyond space and time. The spiritual is limitless, boundless, full of infinite potential. This is the true reality.

Ignorance is what causes our misery. Ignorance is not knowing who we are; it's buying into the limitations of who we are as presented by society, or by the ego. Self-Affirmation helps with this. We can reassure ourselves over and over again of what is real. It's those "I AM" statements that affirm our reality that can help us overcome the misguided sense of lack we often feel. Watch what words follow whenever you say: "I am _____." How are you defining yourself? Differentiate between how you "feel" versus who you are. Rather than saying "I am angry" and taking on the persona of anger – choose instead to say: "I feel angry." Feelings dissipate. You know you'll feel better in a little bit. You don't have to deny your anger, but you don't have to identify with it, either. By doing this, we are persuading our mind to cooperate, to focus on what we want it to focus on. With our intellect, with our thoughts and our words, we can avoid the effect that any distractions or emotions may have on us because we know better. We can rationalize and reason through our problems and see the bigger picture.

RENUNCIATION

Renunciation means to let go, to give up something. We must give up our childhood to become an adult. We give up bad habits to become healthier. Vedanta, and Jnana Yoga, does not tell us to give up the world, or the things of the world. It shows us that we can give up the world as we think it is, to embrace it for what it really is. It is the process of spiritualization, of deification, of seeing everything in the world as holy. We can see God in the trees and the animals. We can see God in our loved ones, and also in everyone.

Renunciation is not about giving up our worldly belongings, it is instead giving up our attachment to them. When we learn to discern between what is real and what is not real, we understand that what we think is real is not really ours at all. It comes and it goes. But what is real, and everlasting, is priceless, and there is plenty of it for all of us. Love, joy, peace, and freedom: These are the real treasures in our lives. These are "things" that we can't put in a jar and sell. These are things we can't describe with a sound, or a symbol. There is no form to them, and yet we understand exactly what they are, and how important they are in our lives.

> *"Of all the discoveries which men need to make, the most important, at the present moment, is that of the self-forming power treasured up in themselves."*
>
> – *William Ellery Channing (1780-1842)*

79

When we give up our attachment to things, it is easier to give up our desires for things. The desire for things keeps us shackled in bondage. We can never get enough, we can never be fulfilled with these objects that aren't real. There's always something newer, greater, bigger, faster. We can't be satisfied and will always be struggling for more. We get caught up in this cycle of wanting and getting that creates a temporary high, and then ultimately leaves us with a lingering emptiness.

Renunciation allows us to give up greed, and selfishness. We can see the big picture, and how all the parts are affected with any action. It becomes important for us to care for ourselves in a way that benefits the whole, the One. It could be as simple as giving up the paper or plastic grocery bags at the store and bringing reusable bags. In so many small ways we can look out for ourselves and our fellow humans and this beautiful planet we share. And then we understand that we're not giving up any "thing" because it's not "ours" to give up in the first place. There's a respect and a deep appreciation that comes with renunciation.

DISCIPLINE

We learn in Jnana Yoga that to obtain knowledge we need to exercise the mind. This is a constant process of learning and using the new tools we are given by putting them into practice. Vedanta explains that there are three criteria for Truth. When only one is present, then this is a partial truth. But when all three are in accordance then we can recognize this as Truth.

1. *Scripture.* Scripture is knowledge that has been learned by others, what has been written down, taught, handed down over the years. It could be in a religious text, a non-fiction book, or in an academic textbook.

2. *Reasoning.* This is knowledge that we come by ourselves by thinking, and figuring out what makes sense to us. We mentally digest what we have read and come to our own conclusions about it. We ask ourselves: Is this reasonable? Do I believe this to be true?

3. *Personal Experience.* This is knowledge that we come by through experience. When we have actual experience then our five senses help us to decide if something is true or not. Personal experience comes in the doing. It's active rather than passive. We know something to be true because we've "been there, done that."

With any given situation we can ask ourselves if these three criteria are present. We don't have to take someone's word for it; we don't have to believe everything we read. And we also don't have to rely on our own intelligence alone. We have access to all kinds of knowledge and wisdom all around us.

"As far as we can discern, the sole purpose of human existence is to kindle a light of meaning in the darkness of mere being."

– Carl Jung

Mental Discipline

It takes mental discipline to control the mind. The mind is susceptible to the ego, and that ongoing conversation it carries on while the ego tries to convince us to look at what the ego feels is important. We have to constantly remind ourselves to use discrimination, to sort out what is real and what is unreal.

It also takes mental discipline to control the senses. As human beings, this is something we can do. Other animals are not as equipped in this kind of discipline as we are. Untrained dogs bark, attack, mount because this is their instinct, and there is little filter there to maintain control. We humans are still susceptible to cravings, and even addictions, because we are so influenced by our senses, but we are capable of learning to have control. It takes maturity to have discipline over the senses. A toddler might not be able to say "no" to a cookie – but as we learn and grow and experience the consequences, we can think things through and decide if we can afford the calories, the sugar, and whatever else comes with that cookie. We can live in the present while considering the consequences that we will face in the future with the decisions we make. So we don't immediately indulge, we give it some thought. A list of questions goes through the brain before we give our answer.

Overcoming Desires

Mental discipline can also help us to overcome our desires. Desire in and of itself is not a bad thing. We can desire world peace, we can desire a more meaningful existence, and we can desire a sense of calm. It's when our desires take us off the path and into the material world that we are led astray. Because a desire for anything that is not real will never be satisfied. No matter how much "stuff" we accumulate it's never enough. What we need to do is to be happy right here and now, with exactly what we have. Desire what you already have, without attachment to it, rather than desiring what you don't have.

Sometimes you need to release old attachments that no longer serve you. Vedanta teaches us to not be possessive. Not being possessive means to not accumulate material objects, to not hold onto toxic relationships, and to not hold on to our past. Every moment is new, and every day holds new promise and opportunities. There is no benefit in hanging on to old "stuff," even if you *think* this is what you want. Jnana Yoga says that we can counter these "false" desires by remaining detached, and remembering the reality of who we really are. One tool to help practice this mental discipline is gratitude. Count your blessings. You might think you have nothing – but this is not the truth. You have everything. You have the sky, the sun, this life. We need to constantly remind ourselves of this. When we realize that we have everything, there is no desire, there is no reason to want for anything.

> *"Don't spoil what you have by desiring what you have not."*
>
> *– Epicurus c. 315 BC*

While mental discipline allows us to control the mind, the senses and our desires, it can also help us with self-control. Mental discipline helps us to be patient, to be tolerant, to maintain our composure in times of stress and difficulty. It's the whole "think before you speak" and "look before you leap" mentality. With this discipline we restrain ourselves, we are not so impulsive or reckless in our thoughts and actions. And this is a good thing! It shows spiritual progress to be careful rather than careless. When we have this mastery over the self, we are not so quick to anger, or judgment.

It takes mental discipline to keep our emotions in check. It's really a habit that we can get into. We can feel the emotions, but it becomes more a matter of observing them, appreciating them, and dealing with them, rather than freaking out, or lashing out. We don't have to cope with the aftermath of our fury or elation. And when we get to that point life is so much easier to handle.

> *"To have ideas is to gather flowers. To think is to weave them into garlands."*
>
> *– Anne-Sophie Swetchine, 1869*

Mental discipline also helps us to observe our own actions. It takes practice to look at our own role in any given situation, rather than blaming, or accusing. We can take responsibility for our actions, as well as our response to any action. It all comes back to us anyway. We're all connected to each other, so how one of us responds will affect how others respond. We can be mindful of our thoughts and actions.

Faith is another practice that requires discipline. Too often when something that we perceive as "bad" happens our brain right away goes to that place of "oh, no" and "now what" and other fearful thoughts. But we can train ourselves instead go to that place of faith – where we observe, calmly, knowing that this is just another event in the play. We think: "This, too, will pass," and "there is a reason behind this."

Mental discipline is not unlike any other kind of discipline. An athlete learns, through training, to control the body. It requires effort, and work, and practice, and the results are evident and even measureable. We marvel at the physical mastery of a ballerina, or a basketball player for example: the strength, the grace, and the balance. These same qualities, mentally, strength, grace, and balance, can be ours with the kind of discipline that is expressed in Jnana Yoga. We can approach this practice as an athlete in training. With the help of our intelligence and understanding we can control the mind. In doing so, we replace ignorance with knowledge.

LONGING FOR LIBERATION

Jnana Yoga says that to attain liberation, or freedom from karma, we have got to want it. Not just "want" this freedom, but long for it. Vedanta says that the degree to which we experience free will over determinism depends on our level of consciousness. The more "awake" we are, the more liberated we are, the more we are free to create the life, and the world, we choose to live in. We have to make liberation our priority, and live our lives every day with this in mind. Our spiritual practice comes into play here. How do we spend our time? What choices are we making? What company do we keep? What foods do we eat? Jnana Yogis understand that these decisions are all a part of our dharma.

> *"There is one quality which one must possess to win, and that is definiteness of purpose, the knowledge of what one wants, and a burning desire to possess it."*

> *– Napoleon Hill*

Meditation is a very effective tool in helping to lead us to liberation. All of the Yogas are in agreement with this, and there is more information on meditation in the Raja Yoga section. There is so much "noise" in the world, so many distractions that take our focus away from our spiritual practices. Meditation helps to put us back on track; it helps to center us so that we can more efficiently and gracefully deal with anything that comes our way during the day. There are many different types of meditation, and you can experiment to find which is best suited to your personality. You may also change it up every once in awhile to keep your practice fresh. Group meditation is especially beneficial, as like-minded people gather and the energy in the room is raised to help everyone feel the peace.

It is important to keep the company of people who understand that spirituality, and ultimately liberation, is a priority. This community support will encourage you to continue with your practice. And the more people you have around you who are doing the same thing, the harder it is for your ego to argue with you that this isn't important.

Attend lectures, take classes, read books, have discussions, bring together people who want to learn. I can personally recommend the classes at The Chopra Center (www.Chopra.com) and the Ayurvedic Institute (www.ayurveda.com). There are also wonderful opportunities to learn at the Life Spa (www.lifespa.com) and you can take online courses, including some of my own, through Daily Om (www.dailyom.com). Other people can be great

WHAT'S YOUR DHARMA?

teachers for us as well. It's not just the people who
are at the front of the class giving instruction; it's
anyone with whom we come into contact. Our relationships bring with them lessons, we just need to be
aware of this so we can learn from them.

"The teacher is no longer merely the-one-who-teaches,
but one who is himself taught in dialogue with
the students, who in turn while being taught also
teach."

– Paulo Freire (1921-1997)

In India there is a tradition of having a guru. This
is someone who is basically an example of what is
possible when you're on the path, and someone who
can show you the way when you get off-course. In the
western world we have teachers, and mentors. Life is
just one big classroom, and we each have something
to offer to our fellow students. There are times in our
lives when we can benefit from having a mentor, and
there are times in our lives when we can benefit from
being a mentor. I'm a Big Sister with Big Brothers Big
Sisters of America. This is a wonderful organization
that matches up kids (Littles) with adults (Bigs) who
can give them some time, attention, and guidance.
Having gone through this experience, I can say that
I have learned so much by extending myself in such
a way. Although I entered into the commitment to
be of service, I quickly found that I was gaining ten-
fold in terms of knowledge, compassion, patience
and understanding. It's a beautiful thing. If you'd

like more information, go to www.bbbsa.org to find a chapter in your area.

> *"Give. Remember always to give. That is the thing that will make you grow."*

> *– Elizabeth Taylor*

Our actions, our daily activities and duties, can be a gauge to see how much we truly long for liberation. Our priorities become very clear when we look at the choices we are making. The body is the vehicle through which we experience liberation, so it is important for us to take care of it. Jnana Yogis study the body, and learn how to help it function optimally. There is a lot to learn, and when we are armed with knowledge, we can make better decisions about our health. We need to eat healthy, wholesome foods, and to exercise. We need to exercise our minds as well, and challenge ourselves intellectually. And we need to take time in silence, through prayer or meditation, to center ourselves spiritually. The body has its own intelligence, and it will tell us what it needs if we just listen. The body is an instrument for our intuition – when we get those "gut feelings" there's a reason, so pay attention.

SELF-KNOWLEDGE

According to Jnana Yoga, this longing for liberation, or the desire for enlightenment, is the first level toward the ultimate goal of transcendence, which is the highest level of Self-knowledge. From there we go through a kind of curiosity, investigating and questioning and figuring out what rings true for us. This is an ongoing process. These levels are not static; we go through them again and again, depending on our mindset and the external factors that are affecting us at the time. There is a state of awareness that we experience in meditation where we actually feel the connection, the Oneness, with everything. This gives us a glimpse of the "real" reality, it is a kind of self-realization. From there we get closer to the direct experience, the direct knowledge of God, or Brahman. We experience non-attachment to the things of the world. And then we even get past the perception of objects to see that they are not real, just an illusion created by the mind. We see the people of the world as our family. And finally we reach transcendence, which is rising above all of the non-real and seeing the Truth, and knowing who we are beyond any labels we wear or roles we play. We see others not just as family – we see others as ourselves.

> *"Knowledge is the annihilation of the separation between me and the other."*
>
> *– Swami Prajnanpad*

Jnana Yoga sums this up by saying that liberation is inevitable, and there are two stages to get there. The first is the movement of consciousness from without, to within. Or we could also say the movement from the focus on the external, to the focus on the internal. We take in wisdom, experience, scripture, and process all of this so that it makes sense to us. We live in a world where our senses are bombarded by stimuli, but we can sort this out, and remain calm amidst the storm. The second stage is the movement of consciousness from within, to without – or from internal to external. Once we are solid in the knowledge of what is real, we now see our place in the world. We see that there is unity and harmony in the midst of what seems to be diversity. This self-knowledge brings us peace, and a sense of joy. It gives us humility as it brings us closer to all the creatures of the world. The veil of illusion is dropped, maya goes away, and we are free.

EXPRESSIONS OF JNANA YOGA

Jnana Yogis have a natural curiosity to their personalities. They are the ones who always want to explore, to investigate, to look further into any situation. They are the ones who ask questions the rest of us hadn't thought of. There is a kind of hunger for knowledge that they are always looking to satisfy. These are people who value intelligence, and who strive for higher education, whether it be through schools or self-taught. They love history, and they love solving puzzles. Jnana Yogis will happily wander the aisles in bookstores and spend hours in museums. You can bet they know their way around a computer, and may have researched the family genealogy online.

You'll find many Jnana Yogis teaching at a university level. And there will be many Jnana Yogis in the classroom as well. They're the serious students, and they usually sit toward the front of the room. Jnana Yogis make good judges, lawyers and mediators because they can often see both sides of an issue, and argue their points sharply. They also make good detectives because they can analyze evidence, and pick up on clues that others might miss. They are very discerning and they can easily sort out what is important. They do very well in the field of science, which allows them to do research and experiment with new ideas and theories. Journalism is an attraction for Jnana Yogis, as in this field they need to organize thoughts and present ideas in such a way that their audience understands what is important to know.

"Reason consists of always seeing things as they are."

– Voltaire (1694-1778)

"I am a Jnana Yogi and my purpose is to know."

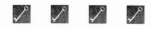

RAJA YOGA
The Path of Meditation

RAJA YOGA
The Path of Meditation

"The phrase 'to meditate' does not only mean to examine, observe, reflect, question, weigh; it also has, in the Sanskrit, a more profound meaning, which is 'to become.'"

–Krishnamurti

MEDITATION AS SCIENCE

Thousands of years ago when the Rishis, the Vedic sages, were writing about the Yogas, Raja Yoga was often referred to as the Yoga of Psychology. In Vedanta, Psychology was known as the science of all sciences. In the western world, we think of psychology as the scientific study of the human mind, and how the mind affects our behaviors. We can apply this understanding to meditation, and see that Raja Yoga is actually a scientific method of finding the Truth, and of experiencing it directly. With the knowledge of this Truth comes freedom, which is the goal of each of the Yogas.

If you find that you are on the path of Raja Yoga, you will experience great insights through introspection. This is your dharma, how you learn and grow. You treasure your private time, and find great peace and joy in the quiet times. Although this may sound very passive, Raja Yogis are quite powerful. When Raja Yogis bring their energy into the world they create a sense of calm and contentment wherever they go.

Science operates very thoroughly and systematically. There are definite procedures and protocol to follow. Scientists make observations, and then generalizations. They study facts, apply scientific principles, and ultimately draw conclusions. Science is a process that works with natural laws, and that has led to amazing discoveries, inventions and technologies that we enjoy today. Like any good scientist, we can use the tools that Raja Yoga provides for us to study the mind, and to acquire the knowledge that we long for.

"Often people attempt to live their lives backwards: they try to have *more things, or more money, in order to* do *more of what they want, so they will be*

happier. The way it actually works is in the reverse.
You must first be *who you really are, then,* do *what*
you need to do, in order to have *what you want."*

– Margaret Young

Raja Yoga explains that the mind has been trained,
since childhood, to focus externally. As children
we play with toys, and as we get older we tend to
want bigger, faster, cooler and more expensive toys.
These toys, the things of the external world, are
distractions. They prevent us from looking within,
from focusing internally. Ah, but the real treasure is
within each of us. We just don't see it because we're
so busy looking everywhere else. Raja Yoga teaches us
how to re-train the mind. It's about paying attention,
and turning the power of the mind back upon the
mind. When we learn to concentrate the power of
the mind we experience all that is possible. The
more concentration we have, the more knowledge
we gain. Raja Yoga is about how to concentrate the
mind, and how to control the mind, so that we can
learn and grow and remember who we really are.

Dr. Maya Angelou is a wonderful example of a
Raja Yogi. She is known as a "Global Renaissance
Woman" and is regarded as one of the great voices
of contemporary literature. She wears many hats,
as a poet, educator, historian, best-selling author,
actress, playwright, civil-rights activist, producer and
director. She has traveled extensively all around
the world, sharing her legendary wisdom. Dr.
Angelou has received over 30 honorary degrees and

is Reynolds Professor of American Studies at Wake Forest University. In her autobiography, *I Know Why the Caged Bird Sings*, she writes: "A bird doesn't sing because it has an answer. It sings because it has a song."

> *"Learn to get in touch with the silence within yourself, and know that everything in life has purpose. There are no mistakes, no coincidences, all events are blessings given to us to learn from."*
>
> – Elisabeth Kubler-Ross

Many times we learn and grow the most when we are faced with adversity. The inevitable problems we encounter in our lives challenge us to reach deeper, to summon our strength, to regain our balance so that we can go on and fulfill our dharma. Challenges can definitely be a distraction that veers us off of our path. Or they can be great lessons for us that teach us how to maneuver our way more gracefully. The approach is up to us. Raja Yoga arms us with tools for the journey.

There is a Zen story about some squashes that were growing on a vine behind a temple. They would often squabble and bicker, and one day a big fight broke out among them. The squashes split into angry groups and created such a commotion that the head priest went outside to scold them. The priest said: "Hey! Settle down Squashes! Why do you fight? Right now, everyone sit and meditate." The priest taught them how to sit straight and still, to close their eyes and be silent. The squashes calmed down and stopped fighting. Then the priest said: "Now everyone put your hand on top of your head." The squashes felt the top of their heads and found that there was something attached. It was the vine that connected each of them all together. "Oh! We have been so foolish!" the squashes said, realizing their situation. "We are actually all connected, living just one life!" From then on the squashes never fought again.

On the path of meditation, we don't need any special instruments, we don't need to go anywhere, or even "do" anything. We just need to "be." And what might sound easy could likely be a challenge at first. We are so used to going and doing and making, putting our attention on the external, that to go within is a foreign concept to us. But it doesn't have to be. Raja Yoga outlines a very specific, scientific approach that anyone can follow.

THE EIGHT STEPS

There are eight steps to follow in Raja Yoga. To make it easier, let's break it down into three basic categories. We can look at the entire process basically like building a house, and Raja Yoga is the blueprint. There's the foundation, and then the structure, and then the interior work, like the wiring and the plumbing, that makes the house come to life.

"There are two mistakes one can make along the road to truth; not going all the way and not starting."

– *The Buddha*

THE FOUNDATION

1. Yama: Truthfulness, Non-Violence

The basic principle of Raja Yoga, which serves as the foundation for this path, is purity. The first step is called "Yama" and this includes having the virtue of truthfulness. Truthfulness means being honest with ourselves, and with other people, in thought, word and deed. We need to have integrity, to do what we say we are going to do. We need to watch ourselves, observe our own behavior. We need to show moderation in our behavior, not overdoing in any particular area. We must not be obsessed with, or addicted to anything.

A part of truthfulness is not claiming something as yours that does not belong to you, so Raja Yoga says we are not to steal, and also we are not to be greedy. We can live life simply and happily, we don't need to possess so many objects. Our load is lighter with fewer possessions. We have less to worry about, less to lose. Think about when you go on a trip somewhere, and you have to live with just what is in your suitcase for a given period of time. It's not so bad, right? It is actually quite freeing!

"We cross the infinite with every step, and encounter the eternal with every second."

– Rabindranath Tagore

Another virtue that is a part of Yama is *ahimsa*, which is non-violence, or non-harmfulness. We need to take care of each other, and of this planet. The easiest way to do that is to do no harm. Harm is not just physical – it can be mental as well. Don't hold on to grudges – when you do you're harming yourself. Let it go. Just a word, or a look, can harm someone, so we must be ever mindful. Deepak Chopra has started a worldwide movement to create peace that starts with each one of us. We can take a vow of non-violence and start by thinking peace. More information is available on the website: http://itakethevow.com/vow. His goal is to get 100 million people to take this vow and by doing so create global change.

Raja Yoga is a very rich practice, and you can see that each step along the way could have many layers of growth within it. To practice ahimsa could vary in meaning to each of us. And the longer we practice Raja Yoga the more deeply we understand and take these virtues to heart. To many yogis ahimsa means that they will not eat meat, because by doing so they are contributing at least in part to the harm of an animal. We have reached the goal of ahimsa when we no longer even have the thought of causing any harm.

"If you see God within every man and woman, then you can never do harm to any man or woman. If you see God in yourself, then you attain perfection."

– The Bhagavad Gita

2. Niyama: Discipline, Contentment, Selfless Service

Niyama is the second step in Raja Yoga and it goes a bit further. It's more than just "not" doing something – it's about having discipline, behaving ourselves, making good choices and being responsible. Rather than just not doing harm, it's about doing good. It's about studying, learning, consciously making the effort to make ourselves better and more pure.

Swasthya is a Sanskrit word that translated means "established in oneself." This is joyfulness, contentment, and perfect health. In our hectic lives it seems that swasthya is elusive. We look for joy outside of ourselves, in our work, or with our relationships, or even with money. We think that more is better, and put our focus too much on the goals ahead of us, without noticing all the beauty that is among us right where we are. Fortunately, we can change our mindsets. Joy is within us! One way we can tap into that joy is with meditation. When we quiet our minds, we release the stresses that have accumulated, and allow the mind and body to get the rest it needs. We can further reap the benefits by supplementing our practice with aromatherapy, herbal teas, warm baths, and massage. It's all a part of taking care of ourselves, of finding that balance that helps us to function optimally. We also need to be mindful of what we put into our bodies. Drink lots of water to cleanse and moisturize the entire system. And eat fresh, nourishing foods. Most importantly, don't postpone happiness. Do what you love to do. Be in a place of gratitude. Spend time with loved ones.

When we are happy with what we have, and with who we are, then we are more peaceful and content. We can guide ourselves toward more spiritual goals and not be distracted with material goals. We can choose to read more spiritually uplifting books and participate in spiritual pursuits.

> *"True happiness… is not attained through self-gratification, but through fidelity to a worthy purpose."*
>
> *– Helen Keller*

"Seva" is a Sanskrit word meaning selfless service. Seva is doing good work, helping others, without attachment, and without any desire for personal gain. It is selfless, a service which is performed without any expectation of result or award for the person performing it. Performing Seva on a regular basis is one way for us to become more aware of our connection with the divine. Just one small act of Seva a day can bring about tremendous spiritual growth.

THE STRUCTURE

Once we have the foundation in place, we can start working on the structure of the building. Raja Yoga says that there are experiences in our lives that have left impressions on us. These impressions are called "samskaras" and they affect our character. We take on the tone of the samskaras, whether they are positive or negative. When samskaras are not good for us, they are kind of like the gutters in a bowling alley. We have gotten into bad habits, so that when we throw the ball, the ball gravitates toward that gutter. It's almost automatic. Of course, when the ball heads down that way then no pins get knocked down, so it doesn't help us win the game. But habits are made, so habits can be broken. Raja Yoga says that we need to counter our bad habits with good habits, over and over again, so that the effects of the old samskaras are lessened. With good habits we can get the bowling ball down the lane all the way and score. We never have to land in the gutter again! Over time, we can even create a little groove that goes right down the center so we get a strike every time. The key is to practice these good habits. And Raja Yoga explains exactly how to do that in the next three steps.

"Our contribution to the progress of the world must, therefore, consist in setting our own house in order."

– Mahatma Gandhi

3. Asana: Perfect Balance in Mind and Body

The postures used in Yoga are called "asana" and this is the third step in Raja Yoga. As we think of Yoga today, as practiced in the various studios around the world, Yoga is an exercise, a way to stay fit and healthy. But it is so much more than that. The word "Yoga" is derived from the Sanskrit root verb *yuj.* which means "to join" or "to unite." It signifies the joining of the individual with the universal reality. It also means the union of the conscious mind with the deeper levels of the unconscious, which results in a totally integrated personality. Just as Ayurvedic practices seek perfect balance in the human body, the yogic ideal of unification is perfect balance or a state of naturalness. Every living being strives toward this ideal, which is described in the Christian religion as "the peace which passeth all understanding." As we begin to search for balance and natural harmony in our own lives, we start to grow on a path that leads to deeper understanding and fulfillment. At such a time we learn that satisfaction comes from something that is found deep within and does not rely on external stimulation. In the sixth chapter of the *Bhagavad Gita*, the textbook of Yoga philosophy, Yoga is explained as meaning a deliverance from the sorrows of this world:

> *When his mind, intellect and self are under control, freed from restless desire, so that they rest in the spirit within, a man becomes a Yukta - one in communion with God. A lamp*

*does not flicker in a place where no winds blow;
so it is with a Yogi, who controls his mind,
intellect and self, being absorbed in the spirit
within him. When the restlessness of the mind,
intellect and self is stilled through the practice
of Yoga, the Yogi, by the grace of the spirit within himself, finds fulfillment. Then he knows
the joy eternal which is beyond the pale of the
senses which his reason cannot grasp. He
abides in this reality and moves not therefrom.
He has found the treasure above all others.
There is nothing higher than this. He who has
achieved it, shall not be moved by the greatest
sorrow.*

Although balance is basic to all existence, it is
often upset. Yoga attempts to restore it through a
threefold path of development: physical, mental,
and spiritual. Yoga teaches that there is no artificial
separation between that the body and the mind.
The goal is to gain control of the body's energy flow
and to direct it in positive, healing ways. Asana is
useful in preparing the body for meditation. Sitting
for an extended period of time requires a flexible
and cooperative body. Physical distress can be
distracting, so by learning to control the body, it is
easier for us to control the mind.

The Indian sage Patanjali, codified the complete system of Yoga asana in the second century B.C. He
said: "The posture of yoga is steady and easy." In the
Yoga Sutras, which remain very important in India
to this day, Patanjali describes eighty-four main Yoga

postures from the thousands then in use. These same postures are basic to the study of Yoga in India today. Sutra in Sanskrit translates to "stitch" as in a thread of knowledge. The Yoga Sutras consist of 195 bits of knowledge that are essentially a guide for living a moral life. They provide a thorough and consistent philosophical basis for yoga, and they also clarify many important concepts in Indian thought.

The sutras are another way for us to get into good habits of thought. The goal of Raja Yoga is to be able to see the Soul, to know the Truth of who we are. Too often we identify with the body, our senses connect us to the world so we think this is who we are. We become attached to the body, the way it looks, feels, and perceives everything around it. Or we may even think that we are the mind, because we have these thoughts that come out of our experiences that say: "I am good" or "I am bad" in judgment. We feel kind and we think we are that, and then we feel anger and we think we are that. The sutras give us "food for thought" – little tidbits of wisdom to contemplate and learn from. There are many different translations and interpretations of these sutras, and we have to form our own ideas and come to our own conclusions as to their meanings.

Focused attention is valued because it helps us in many areas of our lives. The Yoga Sutras of Patanjali break down for us what it takes to achieve this. These are qualities that we can embody, ways of being rather than things to do. Here are a few examples:

Sutras: Qualities to Achieve Focused Attention

-Shraddha: Faith, trust. We need to trust in the intelligence of the Universe and welcome any experiences that come our way. It is about accepting and loving what is, rather than what we think should be.

-Virya: Strength. This is inner strength, fortitude. It is the ability to remain undistracted by disturbances, and to be resilient when things go wrong.

-Smrutti: Memory. When we have certain things learned by memory, whether it is the times tables or our social security number, it gives us more mental energy because we don't have to bother with trying to remember. A good memory allows us to think more clearly and effectively.

-Prajna: Discernment. This is knowing what is real and what is not real. It is understanding where we need to put our attention.

> *"A man is a universe in miniature, and the universe, a giant living body; the cosmos is similar to a large man, and a man is similar to a small cosmos; so say the Sufis."*
>
> *– Kabir*

4. Pranayama: Controlled Energy

The vital energy called *chi* by the Chinese and *ki* by the Japanese is called *prana* in India. Prana is seen to be everywhere and in everything; it is the basic force that animates all matter. In the study of Yoga, the life force, or prana, is closely associated with breathing practices that control and direct this important energy. Freed and able to flow through-out the body, it can stimulate both body and mind; blocked and distorted, it can sap and deplete a person's activities.

Pranayama is really the knowledge and control of Prana. Since it is difficult for us to control the source of all the energy in the universe, we can start learning to control what is nearest to us. The body and mind is what we have to work with. It's as if Prana is the whole ocean, and our own Prana is one wave. We can learn to control our own wave. Breathing exercises are a tool we can use to help us to become aware of our Prana. There are many dif-ferent practices, but each movement of pranayama involves the inhalation, retention, and exhalation of breath. This practice is said to purify the mind, and remove distractions from the mind so that we can concentrate more easily.

Each of the yoga postures is enhanced by the addi-tion of Pranayama. The stretches, breathing tech-niques, and deep-relaxation exercises balance and tone the entire body. They provide an effective method for dealing with today's fast-paced lifestyle and give quick and observable results in relieving stress and tension.

"To grow is to go beyond what you are today. Stand up as yourself. Do not imitate. Do not pretend to have achieved your goal, and do not try to cut corners. Just try to grow."

– Swami Prajnanpad

5. Pratyahara: Self-Restraint, Self-Control

Pratyahara is translated as a "gathering towards oneself" and it is in practice a restraint of the senses. We are so easily distracted, as our senses take our attention away from whatever it is we are supposed to be focusing on. Meditation requires stillness and concentration, so practicing pratyahara is a necessary step towards controlling the senses. The senses constantly take our attention outward, to the external world, away from the inner world. We get uncomfortable sitting in the same position, we hear a phone ring, or we smell dinner cooking and we feel that urge to get up.

Even in our every day lives we are often slaves to the "monkey mind." With technology as advanced as it is making it easier for us to multi-task, we have trouble focusing on one thing at a time. We could be sitting at a desk working, with the TV on, playing Words with Friends on the phone and carrying on a conversation with a group on Facebook all at the same time. The mind is by nature very active, and we tend to go where it takes us. We can't turn it off. But we can learn to control it, to focus, rather than letting it control us.

"Strength does not come from physical capacity. It comes from an indomitable will."

– Mahatma Gandhi

Raja Yoga teaches us that although the mind is active, that is not where we get our intelligence. We get our intelligence from the soul. The mind is the instrument through which we interpret the world. The soul knows the truth. The soul carries higher knowledge. We must calm the mind so that we can access this knowledge. The analogy of a lake is often used to describe how our perception is altered. When the lake is stirred up, it becomes muddy and unclear. We can't see through to the bottom. However, when the lake is calm, the water is crystal clear and we can the bottom easily.

Raja Yoga says that the only way to learn to restrain the senses and to control the mind is through patience and practice. We begin by sitting. I'd suggest turning the phone off and ridding the room of anything that might cause a distraction to make it easier on yourself at first. You can close your eyes, blocking out the sense of sight. You can also use earplugs if you choose. And then just let the mind go. Observe your thoughts. Watch them, rather than acting on them. Imagine them drifting by as if on a cloud. You'll be surprised at how many thoughts come into your mind. But resist the urge to act on them. Use this time to just sit, nothing more. Do this daily, for several days, and you'll see that over time your thoughts begin to subside when you sit. It's as if the mind knows that you won't act on these thoughts during this time so it doesn't bother. Your mind becomes calmer, more prepared for meditation.

"God made the senses turn outwards, man therefore looks outwards, not into himself, but occasionally a daring soul, desiring immortality, has looked back and found himself."

– The Upanishads

THE INTERIOR WORK

Of course, everything leading up to this point has been interior work as well, because the mind and the body are intricately connected. We couldn't only build an outside of a house – by design the inside is there as well. This section of Raja Yoga is specifically about meditation itself as a practice. Most meditators will tell you that it is best to have a teacher guide you when you are learning how to meditate. It's not that you can do it "wrong" but a teacher can direct you so that you start out with good habits and your practice is more fulfilling and fruitful.

There are some basic guidelines that are helpful to follow:

1. Wear loose, comfortable clothing. This helps you to take your attention away from your

body. You don't want to be distracted with a tight waistband.

2. Set aside a special place for meditation. Meditation is a ritual, and after meditating in the same place several times, your body will start to remember the routine and you'll be more likely to settle in. It is nice to have a meditation shawl to cover your lap or shoulders. That way if you are traveling, you can take your shawl with you and it will help to enhance your practice away from home.

3. Meditate at the same time each day. Preferably twice a day. It's a good idea to "bookend" your day with a meditation in the morning and a meditation in the evening. Don't meditate too close to bedtime or you'll be more likely to fall asleep. Although the practice is relaxing, meditation is about "waking up" rather than falling asleep.

4. Plan your meals around your meditation. You don't want to have a full stomach and be busy digesting, or an empty one and hear it growling!

5. Sit comfortably, or kneel, rather than lie down, to avoid falling asleep. You can sit with your back against a chair, keeping both feet on the ground, or you can sit in the traditional cross-legged position.

6. When you have completed your time in meditation, transition slowly back into activity. Open your eyes, look around, feel your body and take some deep breaths.

There are many different types of meditation. You can learn more about them on my website www.psmeditation.com. Meditation is traditionally done in silence, however there are times when guided meditations are particularly helpful. You'll find some downloadable, guided meditations on my site as well.

> *"Meditation is the dissolution of thoughts in Eternal awareness or Pure consciousness without objectification, knowing without thinking, merging finitude in infinity."*

> *– Swami Sivananda*

6. Dharana: Concentration

Raja Yoga explains that there are three stages in meditation. The first stage is concentration, or Dharana. The way to concentrate the mind is to focus it on one particular object, to the exclusion of everything else. The object could be outside the body, such as a flower, or a candle. Or the object could be inside the body, such as the heart center, or the top of the forehead. The idea is to keep the mind still by having it hold only this object, not allowing the senses to give in to distractions, and not allowing thoughts to stray from that object.

*"Meditation can take place when you are sitting
in a bus, or walking in the woods full of light and
shadows, or listening to the singing of the birds, or
looking at the face of your wife or child."*

– Krishnamurti

One tool for accomplishing Dharana is the mantra.
Mantra in Sanskrit means "instrument of the mind."
A mantra's root is a one-syllable sound that carries
no specific meaning. This is different than a word,
which has both sound and meaning. Strung together
as sounds mantras may have many layers of meaning.
We can bring the mantra into the mind, and when
other thoughts interfere, turn our attention gently
back to that mantra.

"Om Mani Padme Hum" (Ohm Ma-Nee Pod-May
Hum) is one of the most prevalent mantras in Tibet.
It is recited by Buddhists, and painted or carved on
rocks, prayer wheels, and wall hangings. This mantra
is known as the mantra of Chenrezi, the Bodhisattva
of Compassion and the protective deity of Tibet.
The practice of the mantra is said to relieve negative
karma, and help rescue us from suffering. The mantra is more powerful when we think of the meaning
behind these six syllables. Om symbolizes transfor-
mation. Mani means the jewel. The Dalai Lama
says: *"Just as a jewel is capable of removing poverty, so the
altruistic mind of enlightenment is capable of removing the
poverty, or difficulties, and of solitary peace. Similarly,
just as a jewel fulfills the wishes of sentient beings, so the
altruistic intention to become enlightened fulfills the wishes*

of sentient beings." Padme means lotus and symbol-izes wisdom. The lotus is a frequent symbol in Vedic philosophy. It is a beautiful flower that grows out of the mud, but is not affected by the mud, indicating the quality of wisdom, which keeps us out of contra-diction. Hum represents inseparability, and purity, which can be achieved with the unity of method and wisdom.

The meaning of this mantra is translated to: *"I surrender to the jewel within the lotus."* When repeated it reminds us of our commitment to spiritual growth, and how, like the lotus, we can ourselves unfold and grow when we reach towards the light.

Dharana is a practice of training the mind to be still and focus. Concentration is like a muscle; we can work it and develop it. Over time it becomes stronger and more sustained. This is why a regular practice of meditation is so important. For our concentration to become, and remain, strong, we must use it.

> *"Nothing contributes so much to tranquilizing the mind as a steady purpose – a point on which the soul may fix its intellectual eye."*
>
> *– Mary Shelley*

Many different distractions may crop up during meditation. We might feel restless, as though we are missing something, or that we should be "doing" something. Many thoughts will come to us with reasons and excuses not to sit and meditate. Emotions may even rise to the surface and make us feel uncomfortable. Rather than try to control these emotions, simply observe them. Watch them. Learn from them. After meditation, it may be helpful to write down what you felt, and any reasons you think those emotions might have presented themselves. In addition, a salt-water bath after meditation helps the body to process the emotions.

7. Dhyana: Meditation

When the mind is able to sustain concentration over a period of time, this is called Dhyana, or meditation. In this step, the seventh in Raja Yoga, a power flows through the mind toward the object of concentration. The meditator does not sense the object itself, but merely the essence of the object. It is as if the object of meditation and the meditator become one. The effort that we dealt with in Dharana ceases, and concentration is easy and natural. In Dhyana the mind does not waver. The meditator does not even think of the process of meditating anymore. We are not aware of time or space.

The calm state of mind that we experience in meditation helps us to handle any stresses or problems that come our way during the day. Meditation helps us to maintain a peace of mind that serves us no matter what happens in the external world.

*"Life finds its purpose and fulfillment in the
expansion of happiness."*

– Maharishi Mahesh Yogi

8. Samadhi: Divine Peace

Finally, in the highest state of meditation, Samadhi,
the meditator becomes lost in the process. Samadhi
means "absorption" and also "divine peace." In
Samadhi the meditator dissolves; the meditator
becomes one with the whole universe. Samadhi is
absolute bliss, or superconsciousness.

When Dharana, Dhyana and Samadhi are all three
practiced together, this is called "Samyama." In
our house analogy, Samyama is like turning on the
light – it is illuminating the Truth. All the work has
been done, and now all that has to happen is that we
flip a switch. And lo and behold, we can see clearly
and confidently.

*"When water joins with water, it is not a meeting
but a unification."*

– Swami Prajnanpad

PERFECTION

Raja Yoga explains that it is our human nature to
strive towards spiritual growth. We can't help it.
There is something inside of us that calls us to seek
the truth, and to seek freedom. We yearn for it, and

because of this, it is inevitable that we will get there. It's not a competition; we each have our own path and our own purpose and our own experiences to go through along the way. There is perfection in where we are headed, and there is perfection right here where we stand in this very moment because everything we have gone through has led us to this place and time. Swami Vivekananda says: "You are the Spirit. That is the first fundamental belief you must never give up. You are the Spirit within you."

EXPRESSION OF RAJA YOGA

Raja Yogis like spending time alone – and they rarely feel alone or lonely. They get caught up in the moment, in the beauty of nature, in the telling of a joke, and forget where they are. They are able to spend long stretches of time working on a project, without noticing that any time has gone by at all, they can be completely involved and immersed in what they are doing.

Raja Yogis might be called daydreamers. They get lost in thought, or non-thought, content to just be without any expectations of themselves or of others. There's no hurry, no rush. Raja Yogis are often called to study religion, and to become monks or nuns.

Artists, musicians and writers are often Raja Yogis. They can draw from the energies around them to create beautiful works. They have easy access to creativity and it flows through them naturally. It's the poet who turns just the right phrase to capture a feeling we thought was beyond words. The Raja Yogi may be the composer whose piano piece makes an audience cry. You'll also find Raja Yogis in nature – challenging themselves to climb higher, closer to the sky, or to dive deeper into unexplored waters. Because Raja Yogis are so gifted at expressing themselves, and at putting into form some of the thoughts, feelings and emotions we all feel, they make wonderful performers and teachers.

> *"In the depth of your hopes and desires lies your silent knowledge of the beyond; And like seeds dreaming beneath the snow, your heart dreams of spring. Trust the dreams, for in them is hidden the gate to eternity."*

> *– Kahlil Gibran*

"I am a Raja Yogi and my purpose is to be."

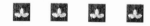

DHARMA
SYMBOLISM

DHARMA
SYMBOLISM

"There is only one thing which can master the perplexed stuff of epic material into unity; and that is, an ability to see in particular human experience some significant symbolism of man's general destiny."

— *Lascelles Abercrombie*

Now that we have read about all four of the yoga paths individually, is easier to understand how all of the paths are really one very wide path as the four intertwine and intersect. Each leads to an awareness of our unity, of our Oneness. Each bring us to self-realization, or enlightenment, or awakening – whatever it is that we choose to call that feeling of complete perfection, of peace of mind, of bliss.

As humans we are multi-faceted, so complex and intricate in design. There are layers to us; there are dimensions to us. There is no one-size-fits-all when it comes to our spiritual growth because we are each so varied in our backgrounds, our priorities, our strengths and challenges. And this is a wonderful thing! It allows us to explore and engage and learn so much from one another.

A peacock shows its colors on the outside. We can literally see the brilliant golds and greens and blues and purples. All of these colors at play together make up one magnificent bird. We humans wear our colors, our passions, our purpose, on the inside. We can't always just look and get the whole picture. It takes some time to get to know our selves and each other. But all those colors are indeed there, expressing through our thoughts and actions. One or two of the colors are more dominant, but all four are there for every single one of us. That is because each path teaches us something, each path guides us towards our purpose and each path IS our purpose. We might say that while the ultimate purpose is awareness, along the way we have four purposes that get us there.

1. To love: Green represents Bhakti Yoga. Green is associated with the heart chakra. Love is associated with the heart symbol, two halves coming together to create one. Bhakti yoga shows us that our purpose is to love. Bhakti Yoga allows us to use our emotions, to feel. By loving others, we love our selves, and we feel our Oneness with the Divine. Green gemstones such as peridot and aventurine help to bring out these qualities and to focus our energy.

2. To serve: Gold represents Karma Yoga. Gold is associated with the sun that serves us all, and brings light to the whole world. Gold is the color of the solar plexus chakra, where we get our "gut" instincts that tell us to take action. Karma Yoga engages us physically, calling us to serve, to work. By giving of our selves, of our time and talents, we are helping humanity, and experiencing our Oneness with the Divine. Citrine and amber are gold colored gemstones that promote optimism and happiness, and help us to find motivation.

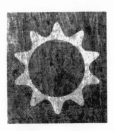

3. To know: Blue represents Jnana Yoga. The symbol of the key represents unlocking the mysteries of life. A key brings us freedom. Blue is associated with the throat chakra, and the third eye chakra, which aids in our communication and intuition. Jnana Yoga stimulates our intellect, and encourages us to think. Through study, thought, and communication we begin to understand our Oneness with the Divine. Turquoise and fluorite are examples of blue stones that help to bring peace to the mind so that we can think more clearly.

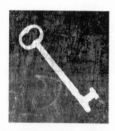

4. To be: Purple represents Raja Yoga. The lotus, with its many petals, is a symbol for meditation, for going within. The lotus flower may have its roots in the mud, but it blooms and grows and brings beauty to the world. Purple is the color of the crown chakra, which connects our physical being to the spiritual realm. Raja Yoga is introspective. It encourages us to be, and to behold. Through silence, through gratitude, appreciation and wonder, recognizing our connection with all of nature, we gain access to our Oneness with the Divine. Amethyst is a gemstone that promotes spirituality and contentment. Iolite encourages self-confidence and success.

Energy Muse makes jewelry that is intended to balance the body through the healing properties of gemstones. To help keep your attention on your dharma, you can wear some of the gemstones. The law of physics explains that thought directs energy and energy follows thought. Each piece of Energy Muse jewelry is designed to help the thoughts of our consciousness connect with our body. Visit the website: www.EnergyMuse.com

In Hinduism, the square is considered to be the perfect shape. A square has four sides, all the same length, and four angles, exactly 90 degrees each. This represents balance, and wholeness. In Vastu, India's science of placement, the perfect floor plan for a house begins with a square, for stability. Four is a significant number. There are four seasons in the calendar year: winter, spring, summer and fall. There are four prime elements: earth, water, fire, and air; as well as four cosmic elements: suns, moons, planets and stars. There are four cardinal directions: north, south, east and west.

In Christianity, there are the Four Gospels: Matthew, Mark, Luke and John. The symbol of the cross is meaningful in many ways in Christian culture. According to sacred geometry, in geometrical terms, the cross is the form of an unfolded cube, and a cube is made up of squares. A cross has four points. It was associated with kings. Many churches were built based on the proportions of the cube or the double-cube. Ancient Egyptians used the square as a symbol of kingship. In Buddhism, the Four Noble Truths are the Buddha's first and principle teaching.

In many cultures, horizontal lines represent the physical realm, or the element of earth, and vertical lines are associated with the spiritual world, or the element of fire. The horizon is a horizontal line separating earth from sky. When a horizontal line and vertical line are put together, as in a cross or a square, this symbolizes two forces that exist in the universe and inside every person as well. We have our need for stability and comfort, our need to feel grounded. And we just as strongly experience our need for growth and change; we are compelled towards evolution.

This is how I came up with the designs for each of the four yogas. When the four squares are put together, they form another, larger square. The colors are from the peacock, the national bird of India. When we see any of these symbols, we can be reminded of the four yogas, and of our purpose here in this space and time.

Now you can proudly wear your dharma! WearLuck has created truly beautiful T-shirts, just for us, using designs based on this dharma symbolism. Check out their website, they have several styles to choose from in each of the four yogas: Bhakti, Karma, Jnana and Raja, and they are all wonderful: www.WearLuck.com.

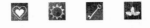

AFTERWORD

"Everyone has been made for some particular work, and the desire for that work has been put into his heart."

– *Djalal ad-Din Rumi*

According to Vedic texts, there are four basic goals of human life. This is something we all have in common. These goals are a fundamental part of our nature, but the attachment to these goals is what causes much of our problems. When we can look at the highest purpose for each of these goals, and not overindulge, we can achieve the bliss that we seek.

-**Kama** means pleasure. In its highest form, this is the pursuit of the preservation of life. When kept in check, kama brings us joy. We eat food that tastes good, as is good for us. We maintain healthy relationships that feed our soul.

-**Artha** means prosperity. In its highest form, this is the pursuit of what we need to thrive, no more and no less. There is no need for waste or greed. We know that accumulation does not bring happiness.

-**Dharma** means purpose, or duty. Dharma is our purpose in life, and we know we are in our dharma when we are doing what we love, and at the same time we are serving others. This is how we use our talents to contribute to society.

-**Moksha** means liberation. In its highest form, this is the pursuit of spiritual growth. When we understand that we are on a spiritual journey in this lifetime, this motivates us further.

> *"Often people attempt to live their lives backwards: they try to* have *more things, or more money, in order to* do *more of what they want, so they will* be *happier. The way is actually works is the reverse. You must first* be *who you really are, then,* do *what you need to do, in order to* have *what you want."*

> *— Margaret Young*

Now that we understand each of the Yogas: Bhakti, Karma, Jnana, and Raja, we can see how they can be used to help us achieve each of the four goals in life, by loving, serving, knowing, and being. Each path has its beauty, and each contributes to our wellbeing.

Wherever you go, whatever you do. know who you are. And know that I am grateful to you for sharing this space and time with me. The Sanskrit greeting "Namaste" means: The divine in me honors the divine in you."

Namaste.

Glossary of Sanskrit Words and Terms

Ahimsa: Non-violence, non-harmfulness in thought, word, and deed.

Artha: Prosperity.

Asana: This is the third of the eight steps in Raja Yoga. Perfect balance. Postures.

Ayurveda: India's "Science of Life."

Bhakta: One who practices Bhakti Yoga.

Bhakti Yoga: The path of love.

Dasya: Loving God as a master.

Dharana: This is the sixth of the eight steps in Raja Yoga. Concentration.

Dharma: Purpose, duty, truth.

Dhyana: This is the seventh of the eight steps in Raja Yoga. Meditation.

Guru: A spiritual teacher.

Hari: One of the Sanskrit names for God, one who attracts all things.

Jnana Yoga: The path of knowledge.

Jnani: One who practices Jnana Yoga.

Kama: Pleasure.

Karma: Work, action, and the effects of that work or action.

Karma Yoga: The path of work.

Madhura: Loving God as our beloved.

Mantra: Sanskrit syllables or sounds that combine into sacred words. Instrument of the mind. A tool used during meditation.

Maya: Illusion.

Moksha: Liberation, freedom.

Namaste: Sanskrit greeting: "The divine in me honors the divine in you."

Niyama: This is the second of the eight steps of Raja Yoga. Discipline.

Om: A mantra in itself. Represents Oneness, the Universal.

Patanjali: Author of the Yoga Sutras, the text of Raja Yoga.

Prana: Life force. Breath. Energy

Pranayama: This is the fourth of the eight steps in Raja Yoga. The control of the life force, controlled energy.

Pratyahara: This is the fifth of the eight steps in Raja Yoga. The control of the senses, self-restraint.

Raja Yoga: The path of meditation.

Rishi: A scholar, sage.

Sakhya: Loving God as a friend.

Samadhi: This is the final step in the eight steps in Raja Yoga. Absolute bliss. Experiencing Oneness.

Samskara: Mental impressions, habits that make up our character.

Samyama: The last three steps in Raja Yoga practiced together: Dharana, Dhayana and Samadhi.

Santa: Peaceful loving.

Seva: Selfless service

Sutra: Stitch, stitch of knowledge.

Swasthya: Established in oneself.

Vatsalya: Loving God as our child.

Viveka: Discrimination.

Yama: The first of the eight steps in Raja Yoga. Truthfulness, nonviolence.

Yoga: To unite, union.

Yogi: One who practices Yoga.

References and Recommended Reading

Adiswarananda, Swami. *The Four Yogas: A Guide to the Spiritual Paths of Action Devotion, Meditation and Knowledge.* Woodstock, VT: Skylight Paths, 2006

Ashley-Farrand, Thomas. *Mantra Meditation: Change Your Karma with the Power of Sacred Sound.* Boulder, CO: Sounds True, 2004

Chopra, Deepak. The Book of Secrets: Unlocking the Hidden Dimensions of Your Life. New York, NY: Random House, 2004

Chopra, Deepak, and Chopra, Gotham. The Seven Spiritual Laws of Superheroes: Harnessing Our Power to Change the World. HarperOne, 2011

DeLuca, Dave. Pathways to Joy: The Master Vivekananda on The Four Yoga Paths to God. Novato, CA: New World Library, 2003

Frawley, David. Vedantic Meditation: Lighting the Flame of Awareness. Berkeley, CA: North Atlantic Books, 2000

Iyengar, B.K.S. Light on Pranayama: The Yogic Art of Breathing. New York, NY: The Crossroad Publishing Company, 2002

Levacy, William R. Beneath a Vedic Sun: Discover Your Life Purpose with Vedic Astrology. Carlsbad, CA: Hay House, 2006

Prabhavananda, Swami, and Isherwood, Christopher. Shankara's Crest-Jewel of Discrimination (Viveka-Chudamani). Hollywood, CA: Vedanta Press, 1947

Satchidananda, Sri Swami. The Yoga Sutras of Patanjali. Integral Yoga Publications, 1990

Vivekananda, Swami. Vedanta: Voice of Freedom. St. Louis, MO: Vedanta Society of St. Louis, 1986

Vivekananda, Swami. Jnana-Yoga. New York, NY: Ramakrishna-Vivekananda Center of New York, 1982

Vivekananda, Swami. Karma-Yoga and Bhakti-Yoga. New York, NY: Ramakrishna-Vivekananda Center of New York, 1982

Vivekananda, Swami. Raja-Yoga. New York, NY: Ramakrishna-Vivekananda Center of New York, 1980

Vrajaprana, Pravrajika. Vedanta: A Simple Introduction. Hollywood, CA: Vedanta Press, 1999

ACKNOWLEDGEMENTS

Back when I was researching my first book I came across Ayurveda, and my life changed forever. Something resonated within me, and I wanted to know more. Deepak Chopra, my friend and mentor, introduced me to Vedanta, and I knew I was home. Thank you to Deepak and to my family at the Chopra Center. What a blessing you are to me!

Barbara Deal is more than an agent and an editor to me; she is a dear friend, and a constant source of inspiration. Thank you to Barbara – for your support and encouragement of my work, and for being the wonderful person that you are.

I am lucky to have a great team to work with at CoffeyTalk – thank you to Brian, Keith, Joel, Rita, Ena, Nancy, Ophelia, Jon, and everyone who works "behind the scenes" to make things happen.

Thank you to my amazing husband, Greg, and our children: Ryan, Freddy, Michaella, Ellen, Brian, and Anika. You are the light of my life!

And much gratitude to my online community of friends – you keep me going! We are all connected and you help me demonstrate this every single day.